ROUTLEDGE LIB
HEALTH, DISE⁄

Volume 11

DISEASE AND
URBANIZATION

DISEASE AND URBANIZATION

Edited by
E. J. CLEGG and J. P. GARLICK

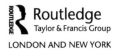

Routledge
Taylor & Francis Group

LONDON AND NEW YORK

First published in 1980 Taylor & Francis Ltd.

This edition first published in 2022
by Routledge
4 Park Square, Milton Park, Abingdon, Oxon OX14 4RN

and by Routledge
605 Third Avenue, New York, NY 10158

Routledge is an imprint of the Taylor & Francis Group, an informa business

© 1980 Taylor & Francis Ltd.

British Library Cataloguing in Publication Data
A catalogue record for this book is available from the British Library

ISBN: 978-0-367-52469-2 (Set)
ISBN: 978-1-032-25316-9 (Volume 11) (hbk)
ISBN: 978-1-032-25318-3 (Volume 11) (pbk)
ISBN: 978-1-003-28266-2 (Volume 11) (ebk)

DOI: 10.4324/9781003282662

Publisher's Note
The publisher has gone to great lengths to ensure the quality of this reprint but points out that some imperfections in the original copies may be apparent.

Disclaimer
The publisher has made every effort to trace copyright holders and would welcome correspondence from those they have been unable to trace.

DISEASE
AND
URBANIZATION

Edited by
E. J. CLEGG and J. P. GARLICK

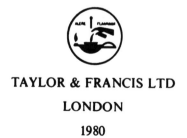

TAYLOR & FRANCIS LTD
LONDON
1980

First published 1980 by Taylor & Francis Ltd, 10–14 Macklin Street,
London WC2B 5NF

© 1980 Taylor & Francis Ltd

Printed and bound in Great Britain by Taylor & Francis (Printers) Ltd,
Rankine Road, Basingstoke, Hampshire RG24 0PR.

British Library Cataloguing in Publication Data

Disease and urbanization. – (Society for the Study of
Human Biology. Symposia; vol. 20 ISSN 0081-153X)
   1. Environmentally induced diseases – Congresses
   2. Medical geography – Congresses
   3. Social medicine – Congresses
   I. Clegg, Edward John   II. Garlick, James Patton
   616.07′1   RB152

ISBN 0-85066-190-0

CONTENTS

PREFACE

In this book we focus attention on selected aspects of disease ecology, which can be resolved into a series of 'contrasts': urban/rural; temperate/tropical; and affluent/poor. In addition to these socio-geographical dichotomies, almost inevitably a further one appears, not an ecological but a nosological one—that between infectious (usually acute) and non-infectious (usually chronic) disease. This dichotomy largely accounts for the temperate/tropical and affluent/poor contrasts and also makes a major contribution to the urban/rural one. Thus, the first group of contributions is concerned largely with infectious disease in rural/tropical/poor societies and the second with the often antithetical combination of chronic disease in urban/temperate/affluent populations.

Not surprisingly, the state of knowledge of the ecology and epidemiology of many diseases falling in the first category is rather poor, although our understanding is constantly increasing. In simple societies living in environments with marked seasonal variation in temperature, rainfall and insolation, environmental pressures fluctuate markedly over the year, and when these variables interact with levels of nutrition varying within or between societies from the more than adequate to the less than inadequate, the complexity of interactions is very great and almost impossible to quantify. However, from the point of view of rational and successful prevention, if it is possible to identify the susceptible links in the chain of transmission of disease from one individual to another, the remaining ecological complexities may be of only minor importance, especially where transmissions can be reduced below critical levels by relatively simple control measures. Thus, for many of these diseases the importance of such simple measures as, for example, satisfactory levels of nutrition, adequate supplies of good water, and improved standards of hygiene, both personal and in food preparation, seem to be of the greatest importance. Where disease is vector-borne, the eradication or at least the control of vectors gives hope for the future, providing that the basic necessity is met of an adequate administrative and educational infrastructure on which can be based effective programmes of preventive medicine.

Thus for the first group of diseases, problems are often identifiable, but very difficult although not impossible to solve. For the second group, however, the identification of problems is often not well advanced. While for the first group the passage of time, with increase in knowledge and improvement in standards of living, can be expected to change things for the better—a view borne out by previous experience in present-day developed countries during their period of rapid economic development—with the second group the reverse situation appears to be the case. Many of the diseases discussed (chest disease, cardiovascular disease) appear to be diseases of affluence—or rather of relative inaffluence in affluent societies. Others, cancer especially, might be regarded as inevitable concomitants of increasing life expectation. While this particular interpretation remains true in general, there is little hope of progress unless it can be partitioned into more manageable components (inherited susceptibility; general or specific environmental stresses (occupational, nutritional); etc., etc.). The identification of specific aetiological factors is no easy matter, yet for many of these conditions specific, 'one-disease', factors may be very important; hence single measures to effect environmental amelioration can be expected to influence only a limited number of diseases. The net result seems to be that despite the enormous human and financial resources being poured into research into, for example, coronary disease and cancer, major advances are dearly bought. Furthermore, affluence, with its emphasis on self-gratification, constantly impedes the implementation of control measures based on ecological and epidemiological evidence even when, as in the association between smoking and a variety of chronic lethal diseases, this evidence is incontrovertible.

For all these reasons the tone of the contributions will be seen to be realistic rather than optimistic. For the infectious diseases, the relative ineffectiveness of malaria eradication programmes in certain ecological conditions, the 'new' (or at least newly recognized) diseases such as dengue haemorrhagic fever, the lethal combination of inadequate diet and infection—all these indicate the necessity firstly for further ecological and epidemiological investigation, but above all for adequate basic health care, in both the cities and rural areas of poor tropical countries. Yet the way ahead seems in many cases reasonably clear; too often what is lacking is the economic ability to follow it.

For the chronic diseases, the outlook is the same—somewhat gloomy, yet with rays of hope occasionally appearing. The progressive identification of specific environmental carcinogenic agents seems to be of potentially great value; the recent reduction in mortality from ischaemic heart disease suggests that the adaptive process (but to what?) may already have begun. For chronic lung disease, general environmental amelioration (smoke-free zones) and individual education (reduction in smoking) should produce good results. In general, one might draw from these papers the conclusion that solutions to many of the problems of disease in urban communities, if not in sight, are not far over the horizon. Implementing them, though, will involve enormous expense and/or major changes in some of the personal habits which are the very hallmarks of affluence.

Thus the tone of this volume is very practical. Given its theme, this could hardly be otherwise. At some points, the objective study of man and the study of the problems he faces in the various ecosystems of which he forms a part come together. This is one of these points.

The organizers and the Society are most grateful to Messrs. Pfizer Ltd., Upjohn Ltd. and the Ciba Foundation for financial assistance. Dr D. A. J. Tyrrell, C.B.E., F.R.S. was most helpful in discussions on the design of the symposium.

ECOLOGICAL FACTORS
IN DENGUE
HAEMORRHAGIC FEVER

W. W. MACDONALD

Department of Entomology, London School of Hygiene and Tropical Medicine

IN addition to malaria, which in some countries, such as India, is an urban as well as a rural problem, there are two widespread and serious mosquito-borne infections in urban communities in parts of the developing world. These are bancroftian filariasis and dengue haemorrhagic fever. Whereas filariasis has been recognized for some hundreds of years and the general features of its epidemiology have been understood since early in this century, dengue haemorrhagic fever presents a relatively new problem. It was only in 1954, during an epidemic in the Philippines, that the infection was recognized as a distinct entity, although retrospective case detection studies have revealed probable earlier transmission. In 1956 a dengue aetiology was established, and in the following years, each of the four types of dengue virus has been isolated during outbreaks.

Following the 1954 outbreak in the Philippines, primary outbreaks were reported in 1958 from Thailand, in 1960 from Singapore, in 1962 from Malaysia, in 1963 from Vietnam and Eastern India, in 1969 from Indonesia, in 1970 from Burma, and in 1972 there was an outbreak on Niue Island in the South Pacific. In most countries there have been recurring outbreaks, and Thailand in particular has suffered severely, with epidemics every year without exception for the past 20 years (Table 1). Dengue haemorrhagic fever has been associated primarily with urban populations, but in Thailand, although the early outbreaks were almost limited to Bangkok, there has been a steady

TABLE 1.   Reported cases of, and deaths from, dengue haemorrhagic fever in Bangkok (including Thonburi) and in all of Thailand.

	Greater Bangkok			All Thailand		
	Cases	Deaths	% Deaths	Cases	Deaths	% Deaths
1958	2 418	240	9·93	2 706	296	10·94
1959	124	15	12·10	160	21	13·12
1960	1 742	59	3·39	1 851	65	3·51
1961	481	23	4·78	561	36	6·42
1962	4 185	216	5·16	5 947	308	5·18
1963	1 657	144	8·69	2 215	173	7·81
1964	5 403	278	5·15	7 663	385	5·02
1965	1 994	59	2·96	4 094	193	4·71
1966	3 046	52	1·71	5 816	137	2·36
1967	834	8	0·96	2 060	65	3·16
1968	1 631	21	1·29	6 430	71	1·10
1969	2 199	19	0·86	8 670	109	1·26
1970	577	19	3·29	2 767	67	2·42
1971	1 092	10	0·92	11 540	308	2·67
1972	2 475	9	0·36	23 786	682	2·87
1973	1 509	22	1·46	8 280	315	3·80
1974	1 068	24	2·25	8 160	328	4·02
1975	1 778	4	0·22	17 767	438	2·47
1976	1 441	13	0·90	9 616	359	3·73
1977	4 235	18	0·43	38 678	746	1·93

spread through the country into townships and villages, and every province in the country has now experienced the infection. In 1974 in Malaysia one of the most severely affected areas was rural western Johore.

The principal vector has almost always proved to be *Aedes aegypti*, but *Ae. albopictus* is sometimes a secondary vector and in the Niue Island outbreak *Ae. cooki* may have been involved, with or without *Ae. aegypti*.

Outbreaks vary in severity both between years and between seasons. In Thailand, the major epidemics were for a time biennial, and this rhythm was particularly evident from 1958 to 1968, when there were peaks in the reported cases during the even years, but in recent years the pattern has been disrupted and 1975 and 1977 had most severe outbreaks (Table 1). A biennial pattern was also clear in Burma, where 1000 to 2500 cases were reported during 1970, 1972 and

1974 and much lower numbers in the intervening years. No satisfactory explanation of this pattern has been proposed. Where there is a pronounced wet season, as in Thailand and Burma, there has usually been a positive correlation between this season and the outbreaks. However, the correlation has not been exact, and significant numbers of cases have been reported at all other times of the year. In Hue, Vietnam, there was an outbreak during the dry season of 1973, and in that case it was thought that an increased number of *Ae. aegypti* were present owing to the increase in the number of water storage containers available for breeding.

In all outbreaks of dengue haemorrhagic fever, children have been most affected. In Bangkok during 1962–65, the median age of children hospitalized was 3 years 10 months. Later, during 1971–73, there was a shift to 5 years 7 months. Where suitable treatment facilities are available, the case fatality rate has fallen to 2 to 5 per cent, and in Bangkok, where medical staff have most experience of the infection, the rate has been reduced in recent years to less than 1 per cent, as compared with rates of about 10 per cent during the outbreaks in the 1950s (Table 1).

The prevention of outbreaks of dengue haemorrhagic fever is dependent at present on control of the vector *Ae. aegypti*. There is no alternative. To control *Ae. aegypti* we need first of all a substantial knowledge of its ecology on which control strategy can be planned, and, secondly, an acceptable means of attacking one or other stage of the life-cycle. We now have a relatively thorough understanding of the mosquito; we now have satisfactory means of attacking both the aquatic immature stages and the adults; but, perhaps paradoxically, we have no immediate prospect of preventing outbreaks. The reason for this pessimistic outlook centres in part around the habits of the people in affected areas, around their beliefs, and sometimes prejudices, and around their lack of appreciation of how essential is the part that they must play before vector control can be achieved. But the administrators and health officials also have heavy responsibilities, and the means by which effective co-operation of health workers and the public can be created need examination and definition.

In the remainder of this paper, the near total dependence of *Ae. aegypti* on man will be demonstrated and our current knowledge on some facets of its ecology will be outlined. Consideration will then be given to aspects of human behaviour which favour the mosquito in order to enquire whether and how changes in man himself could lead to the control of dengue haemorrhagic fever.

Vector Ecology in Relation to Transmission

Ae. aegypti has long been established as a most efficient vector of dengue (and of yellow fever). Its origins are the forests of Africa, where feral populations can still be found, and it has spread outwards into villages and towns first within tropical Africa and subsequently through the warmer regions of the Americas and of Asia and as far as Australia and the South Pacific. The spread has followed the lines of human communications, especially by road, by sea and by rail.

In South-east Asia, survey records show that *Ae. aegypti* at the beginning of the century was primarily a coastal species and that incursions into inland towns and villages have been relatively recent. Even within the past 20 years in Malaysia, the available records point clearly to an inland spread and consolidation of populations. For example, Macdonald (1956) reported three surveys in each of three inland villages, Rembau, Chengkau and Kota, during a period of 20 months from May 1954. In Rembau the proportions of houses with *Ae. aegypti* larvae were 20, 10 and 20 per cent, in Chengkau the figures were 5 per cent, zero and 5 per cent, and in Kota no larvae were found at any of the three surveys. Some 20 years later *Ae. aegypti* was found in approximately half the houses in all three villages, which were situated a few miles apart. There are now few, if any, towns in Malaysia without *Ae. aegypti*, and the same may be true also of villages. During the period 1971–74, staff of the Institute for Medical Research in Kuala Lumpur surveyed 152 towns and villages throughout peninsular Malaysia and, except for 10 villages, *Ae. aegypti* was present in every locality visited (Cheong Weng Hooi, personal communication). In 1970, Macdonald and Rajapaksa (1972) surveyed the distribution and relative prevalence of *Ae. aegypti* in Sabah and recorded a number of areas where it was absent, More recent, unpublished reports give evidence of new foci in several of these areas, notably in the capital town, Kota Kinabalu.

Three adaptations have favoured *Ae. aegypti* in its spread from Africa. First, the species has become strongly domestic and anthropophilic, although hosts other than man, including household animals, will serve as a blood source if the need arises. Second, instead of the ancestral tree-hole, the females now preferentially select man-made containers for egg-laying, such as water jars and drums, discarded tyres, flower vases and tin cans. Third, the eggs, after being laid, may remain for weeks or months in diapause before hatching; this feature is common to aedine mosquitoes, and it has evolved to enable forest-dwelling species to survive in the egg stage through dry seasons when natural containers such as tree-holes dry up.

Larval ecology

The principal larval habitats are man-made containers, and it is not uncommon to find in cities such as Bangkok or Jakarta several breeding-places per household, and in some houses there may be 10 or more. Two indices are commonly used to express the prevalence of *Ae. aegypti* in an area: the *Ae. aegypti* premise index and the Breteau index. The first indicates the percentage of houses with positive *Ae. aegypti* habitats, the second denotes the number of positive habitats per 100 houses. Surveys in South-east Asia of shophouses or of low-income districts often reveal premise indices of 70 to 80 per cent or higher, and Breteau indices of 200 to 300.

The larval habitats are, of course, not of equal importance in their contribution to the adult population. Some kinds of container support larger numbers of larvae than others, and the relative numbers of different kinds may vary both between areas and between seasons or years. It is generally not very difficult to define the distribution and relative prevalence of different habitats, but it is less easy to estimate the contribution which each type makes to the adult population. In low-income areas of Rangoon, the most productive habitats are probably 44-gallon metal drums which are used widely for water storage; in Bangkok, on the other hand, earthenware jars are by far the most prolific, whilst in Jakarta the most important are perhaps the indoor concrete tubs used for storing water for bathing.

The relative abundance of different habitats also varies at a local level. In Malaysia, for example, ant-traps or anti-formicas might account for nearly one-third of positive habitats in shophouses and urban slum areas, whereas in rural Malay houses ant-traps are seldom used. However, with the increased usage of refrigerators throughout the country, the prevalence of food storage cupboards with their legs in water-filled ant-traps may be declining.

In Bangkok, Tonn *et al.* (1969) studied larval habitats in 14 localities at three different times of the year and showed that almost all the differences between localities, including kinds and numbers of containers, and their location indoors or outdoors, were highly significant. The same authors looked at the differences between seasons, and they concluded that in Bangkok, although there were minor seasonal shifts in the type of favoured habitat, the fluctuations in larval populations did not seem to be much greater than 15 per cent between the cool, the warm and the wet seasons.

The most important measurement to be derived from studies of the larval habitat is the output of adults. It is also one of the most difficult to estimate. The output from a class of containers depends on the number of containers, the number of eggs laid in them, the survival rate through the immature stages to the pupal stage, and the emergence rate from the pupae. A few studies have been made, and in Bangkok, for example, Southwood *et al.* (1972) estimated that in a small study area of 0·53 ha there was a mean daily emergence throughout the year of about 77 adults from the principal habitats. The most productive sources were water-jars, which contributed 71 per cent of the adults, although the probability of an egg laid in a jar reaching the adult stage was only 0·012. The two other major habitats were the plates on which flower-pots rested and ant-traps, which contributed 26 per cent and 3 per cent, respectively, to the adult population. In these two kinds of container, the probabilities of an egg giving rise to an adult were 0·135 and 0·019, respectively. From such ecological studies, workers in Bangkok estimated in 1968 that about 800 000 containers supported *Ae. aegypti* in the city and that some 1·9 million adults were emerging each day.

The studies in Thailand have made it possible to define quickly, though approximately, the most productive habitats in any given area, and they have shown that treatment or elimination of only one or two classes of container might reduce the *Ae. aegypti* population by 70 to 80 per cent or more. However, it is not yet possible to define accurately the level of reduction required to prevent virus transmission. The experience of workers in Brazil, where in the past urban yellow fever was transmitted by *Ae. aegypti*, has led to a premise index of 5 per cent being regarded as the level below which transmission would be prevented. The attainment of this level is not easy, but it can be achieved.

Adult ecology

Ae. *aegypti* control programmes generally concentrate on the immature stages and their habitats, but studies on the adults have not been neglected. The most important parameters relating to disease transmission are the numbers of females, their survival rate, the frequency of blood-feeding, and their dispersal pattern. Since the adults bite by day and rest indoors, it is fairly easy to measure relative differences in populations both by time and by place by means of standardized biting or resting catches, and for many purposes the information gained is adequate. For example, seasonal fluctuations can be followed and the effects of temperature or rainfall might be inferred. It is much more difficult to estimate population numbers in absolute terms to provide a figure for the number of mosquitoes per hectare, or per village, or per house. Nevertheless, techniques to give such information are available, and one method, the mark–release–recapture method, has been applied in Bangkok (Sheppard *et al.*, 1969). In that city a study was begun in 1966 to test the currently held view that outbreaks of dengue haemorrhagic fever occurred during the wet season because the numbers of vectors increased at that time. This view was a plausible one, and it was based on the assumption that during the wet season many miscellaneous outdoor containers collected rainwater and so provided a greatly increased number of breeding-places for Ae. *aegypti*. However, general observations in many districts of Bangkok revealed that outdoor containers, other than water-jars, were not common, and, moreover, large numbers of water-jars containing *Aedes* larvae could be found at all seasons of the year.

It was against this background that a mark–release–recapture experiment was begun to measure a population in a small study area of 0·53 hectares and to monitor the numbers more or less continuously for a year. The results, in summary, showed that although there were changes from time to time in the population size, these changes were not correlated in any simple way with either temperature or rainfall. There was an increase during the wet season, but the increase was not pronounced.

Any changes in mosquito daily survival rates affect the population size, so survival rates were estimated throughout the year from the mark–release–recapture data. The estimates revealed no significant differences between months, although there were, as expected, differences between the sexes.

Measurements were also made of the distances and directions moved by marked mosquitoes, and, under the restrictions imposed by the small size of the study area, no significant differences were observed between months.

The frequency of blood-feeding by the vector is clearly most relevant to disease transmission. It is often assumed that a mosquito will feed, rest for 2 to 3 days while the eggs develop, then, after oviposition, feed once again. In the Bangkok study, a record was kept of the condition of every female caught throughout the year — whether unfed, fully-fed, semi-gravid or gravid — and the hope was that by recapturing individuals on several occasions the feeding and egg-laying pattern would be established. However, there was no simple or uniform pattern and mosquitoes recorded on one day as semi-gravid, and with sufficient blood remaining to allow full maturation of the eggs, might be recaptured on the following day distended with fresh blood. This is an important feature of *Ae. aegypti* ecology, which had been reported earlier in Malaysia (Macdonald, 1956), and confirmed subsequently elsewhere in Thailand (Gould *et al.*, 1970). In the latter study, on an island in the Gulf of Thailand, 33 to 58 per cent of *Ae. aegypti* taken during monthly biting collections were gravid. Gravid individuals of a vector of lesser importance, *Ae. albopictus*, were also taken biting, but the monthly proportions in this species were only 6 to 34 per cent. This avidity for blood, even when the blood is apparently not necessary for survival or for egg development, may go some way towards explaining how relatively low populations of *Ae. aegypti* can maintain transmission of viral infections.

It did not prove possible in Thailand to relate discrete outbreaks of dengue haemorrhagic fever with any individual feature of the ecology of *Ae. aegypti*. It seemed from the studies in Bangkok that there was a sufficient population of the mosquito, living long enough and biting often enough, to allow transmission at any time of the year. Observations and studies in Malaysia and Indonesia would lead to the same conclusion for those countries.

Human Ecology in Relation to Transmission

From what has been said of the nature and distribution of the larval habitats of *Ae. aegypti*, it is clear that dengue haemorrhagic fever is a 'man-made' disease. Elimination of the habitats provided by man would stop transmission. Unfortunately those containers which are responsible for most of the adult production are least easily removed, i.e., the earthenware jars, the drums and the cement storage tanks. The frequency of occurrence of these habitats is, in part, related to the local water supply. In many urban districts of developing countries, a piped water supply is often inadequate. There may be periods of the day when the supply is interrupted, so that householders are obliged to store water. In many low-income areas, the people depend on communal standpipes, and each house usually has an adjoining drum to collect rainwater. Even in districts with an apparently satisfactory supply to individual houses, rainwater may be collected and stored for drinking and cooking because it tastes 'sweeter' than the piped water.

Part of the increase in urban mosquito populations, and in mosquito-borne infections, is the result of the unplanned growth of towns and cities. In developing countries the urban human populations have been growing more than twice as fast as those in the more developed lands, and there has been no appropriate increase in water supplies or waste disposal systems. Under such circumstances no blame can be attached to the householders for storing water. In many rural areas of South-east Asia, there is no piped water supply and there is complete dependence on well-water and rainwater. Storage containers are therefore essential.

However, both in urban and in rural areas, there is often an excess of containers, many of which have accumulated over the years and some of which, like broken jars and discarded car tyres, are quite valueless. And it is not only in the poorer communities that these conditions are found. Many sophisticated households with large and well-kept gardens have an unnecessarily large number of jars with water for garden use. There are significant differences between races in their usage and acquisition of jars. In Malaysia, for example, Chinese households, with or without a piped water supply, always seem to have a surplus of storage jars, sometimes ornate and attractive, but often unnecessary. In Malay communities, on the other hand, the presence of storage containers is more directly related to the standard of the water supply. Indian households generally have few jars, and quite commonly, in the absence of piped water to the house, there is only one, which is refilled daily from a communal standpipe.

The problem containers fall into three main classes: those which are maintained for essential water storage; those which are unnecessary, and are often without value, and which could be removed; and those which, like ant-traps and flower vases, could easily be kept free of mosquito larvae by the householder. It is the first group which presents the greatest challenge. In many cases it is not helpful to use lids to prevent mosquito breeding. Lids are usually ill-fitting, and their use may even be beneficial to *Ae. aegypti*. It was shown in Jakarta that jars with lids were more likely to contain larvae than those without. It is not realistic in areas with a poor water supply to propose regular emptying and cleaning of water storage containers. The only remaining choice is to add to the water an agent, either chemical or biological, which will kill immature mosquitoes, or to embark on a long and expensive spraying campaign with insecticides against the adults.

The most effective agent in current use is the larvicide temephos, an organophosphate compound whose safety and efficacy have been demonstrated on numerous occasions. However, it is seldom easy to persuade householders to accept what might be regarded as a contaminant in their water. A common post-treatment reaction is that the housewife empties and rinses the treated jar, and while this may remove the larvae, a new population can be expected a few days later. Although there generally seems less objection to the treatment of large, immovable storage containers, many people — perhaps most — would rather accept the introduction of fish or predacious dragonfly nymphs.

Effective control of *Ae. aegypti* demands the co-operation of the public, and the degree of co-operation achieved depends on education and persuasion and, in many situations, on legislation. Without an education programme, it is difficult to persuade a householder that his water jar with a few dozen larvae must be treated with insecticide while his blocked drain outside, breeding thousands of *Culex* mosquitoes, is ignored. And without legislation to support him, the health worker will often have little success in persuading a factory owner to dispose of discarded motor-car tyres in his yard.

It is unfortunately true that the only successful control programmes have been those in which participation of the public could be enforced by legislation. The two notable examples are from Brazil and Singapore. However, Brazil had the threat of urban yellow fever as an incentive, Singapore had the advantage of having a relatively small population and limited area to administer, and both had well-trained and efficient staff. In most countries of South-east Asia, legislation relating to domestic mosquito breeding would be well-nigh impossible to enforce. Health workers in vector control are too few in number for any prospect of attaining the required standard of supervision and inspection. Means must therefore be found to persuade the people themselves to accept willingly a responsibility for vector control. How this is to be done is the most difficult question facing us today.

Responsibility rests not only with the householder. It is shared by everyone employed on health problems, from the politician to the mosquito scout. Several years ago, at a meeting in Washington, Audy (1972) illustrated how, having created many of his vector-borne disease problems, man was often actively resistant to changes which would lead to their solution. He examined the problems which can arise within and between the groups who have responsibilities in health programmes — the politician and the administrator, the technologists and their field teams, and the householders. He also made the point that although we have large numbers of people trained and experienced in the technical and scientific aspects of vector control work, we have very few trained and experienced in understanding and influencing people. More recently, Gillett (1975) has emphasized the same deficiency, and he made a strong plea for a substantial investment into the study of man himself in relation to mosquito-borne infections. He rightly argued that we know a very great deal about the vectors and about the infections they transmit, but that we have made no real effort to study the behaviour of man and how it may be changed.

The lack of success during the past 20 years in preventing outbreaks of dengue haemorrhagic fever strengthens this argument. The studies made on *Ae. aegypti* during this century would fill many volumes, and we have several means available for reducing populations to low levels, but we have no idea of which methods are acceptable to people in different circumstances, nor of how householders of different nationalities, customs and beliefs might be persuaded to assist their health workers in achieving vector and disease control, and, worst of all, we have made little or no effort to find out. It is difficult to avoid the conclusion, therefore, that infections such as dengue haemorrhagic fever will continue to recur and spread until studies of vector management are supplemented with studies of man management.

Acknowledgement

I am grateful to Dr. Sujarti Jatanasen of the Ministry of Public Health, Thailand for providing some of the data on dengue haemorrhagic fever cases.

References

AUDY, J. R. (1972) Aspects of human behaviour interfering with vector control. In *Vector control and the recrudescence of vector-borne diseases*, pp. 67–82. Washington, D.C.: Pan American Health Organization Scientific Publication no. 238.

GILLETT, J. D. (1975) Mosquito-borne disease: a strategy for the future. *Science Progress, Oxford*, **62**, 395–414.

GOULD, D. J., MOUNT, G. A., SCANLON, J. E., FORD, H. R. and SULLIVAN, M. F. (1970) Ecology and control of dengue vectors on an island in the Gulf of Thailand. *Journal of Medical Entomology*, **7**, 499–508.

MACDONALD, W. W. (1956) *Aedes aegypti* in Malaya. II: Larval and adult biology. *Annals of Tropical Medicine and Parasitology*, **50**, 399–414.

MACDONALD, W. W. and RAJAPAKSA, N. (1972) A survey of the distribution and relative prevalence of *Aedes aegypti* in Sabah, Brunei and Sarawak. *Bulletin of the World Health Organization*, **40**, 203–209.

SHEPPARD, P. M., MACDONALD, W. W., TONN, R. J. and GRAB, B. (1969) The dynamics of an adult population of *Aedes aegypti* in relation to dengue haemorrhagic fever in Bangkok. *Journal of Animal Ecology*, **38**, 661–702.

SOUTHWOOD, T. R. E., MURDIE, G., YASUNO, M., TONN, R. J. and READER, P. M. (1972) Studies on the life budget of *Aedes aegypti* in Wat Samphaya, Bangkok, Thailand. *Bulletin of the World Health Organization*, **46**, 211–226.

TONN, R. J., SHEPPARD, P. M., MACDONALD, W. W. and BANG, Y. H. (1969) Replicate surveys of larval habitats of *Aedes aegypti* in relation to dengue haemorrhagic fever in Bangkok, Thailand. *Bulletin of the World Health Organization*, **40**, 819–829.

FROM MALARIA ERADICATION
TO MALARIA CONTROL

L. J. BRUCE-CHWATT

Wellcome Museum of Medical Science, London

MALARIA has a major place among the endemic tropical diseases. It has been estimated that 20 years ago the annual incidence of the disease was of the order of 250 million cases, with 2·5 million people dying of malaria every year.

Soon after the Second World War, the newly born World Health Organization recognized that malaria not only killed more people than any other disease, but also interfered with the development of agriculture and growth of industry in the tropics. The intensive control methods carried out in some western countries produced excellent results, but could not be easily applied in many tropical areas. The advent of DDT presented the world with a new method of interrupting the transmission of infection by attacking the mosquito vector during its epidemiologically most important stage when it feeds on man in his dwellings.

The epidemiological concept of the interruption of malaria transmission by insecticide spraying is simple. After taking her blood meal, the female anopheline mosquito generally rests on a nearby indoor surface for several hours while the blood is digested and the batch of eggs matures. The female mosquito feeds every 2 to 3 days and the malaria parasite, after being ingested with the blood, requires at least 10 to 12 days for its full development to an infective stage. Spraying all inside wall surfaces of human dwellings and other domestic shelters with a long-lasting insecticide like DDT would therefore create conditions in which a substantial proportion of anopheles would be killed before they could transmit malaria.

It soon became obvious that the eradication of malaria did not require the total elimination of all the vectors, and several examples of successful campaigns (Italy, Cyprus, Greece, Guyana, Puerto Rico, and Venezuela) were most impressive. It appeared that the widespread use of DDT and other residual insecticides for indoor spraying was the most reliable, feasible, and economical method for the interruption of transmission (the attack phase), especially in rural areas. In the next phase of the eradication programme (the consolidation phase), the remaining foci of infection could be detected by proper surveillance and eliminated by distribution of antimalarial drugs and local application of insecticides.

The eradication programme has been defined as an operation aimed at stopping the transmission of malaria and eliminating the reservoir of infected cases in a campaign limited in time and carried to such a degree of perfection that, when it comes to an end, there is no resumption of transmission.

This simplified description of the principle of malaria eradication gives no idea of the operational complexity of a large-scale programme. Few other public health endeavours need such careful planning, efficient administration, adequate financing, and detailed evaluation. The worldwide programme of malaria eradication was formally endorsed by the Eighth World Health Assembly in 1955 and in 1957 the World Health Organization took over the co-ordinating activities and the provision of technical assistance. The concept of malaria eradication was accepted by all the member governments of the World Health Organization. Previous control programmes were converted to eradication, and eradication programmes were initiated in all malarious countries in the Americas and Europe, and in the majority of countries in Asia and Oceania. But only pilot projects were attempted in Africa.

What is the situation today after nearly 25 years? According to the latest reports for 1976, malaria has been eliminated from the whole of Europe, most of the Asian part of the USSR, several countries of the Near East, most of North America including the whole of the USA, most of the Caribbean, large areas of the northern and southern portions of South America, Australia, Japan, Singapore, Korea and Taiwan. There is little official information about China, but it seems that malaria has been virtually eliminated from most of that country. A recent (1976) assessment of progress during the past two decades (in

TABLE 1. Progress of anti-malaria programmes between 1957 and 1976.

Location	Population (million)	
	1957	1976
Areas of the world with anti-malaria programmes in various phases	789	1697
Areas without anti-malaria programmes	421	352
All previous and present malarious areas	1210	2048

terms of population protected) shows (Table 1) that malaria eradication has been achieved in areas with a population of 436 million, while extensive control was in operation in areas inhabited by 1256 million. These two figures together represent some 83 per cent of the population of the originally malarious areas. However, the remaining 17 per cent of the unfinished task represents 352 million people in areas without any antimalaria measures, and the bulk of them are in tropical Africa. It is likely that the above figure is rather an underestimate and that a truer number is close to 500 million. Be this as it may, the present risk of malaria infection still exists in parts of the world inhabited by 1612 million people, over the major areas of the developing world. These overall results are of great interest: they justify the original concept and yet show that under some conditions it cannot be pursued to a successful conclusion.

In African countries south of the Sahara, malaria is responsible for about 10 per cent of annual deaths of infants and children below the age of 14 years. These estimates of mortality and morbidity are no more than informed guesses, because of the well-known shortcomings of statistical data in that part of the world. The most striking feature of the disease in tropical Africa is its high endemicity with hardly any seasonal changes; thus, the individual is infected at an early age and is subjected to repeated infections throughout his life. The toll of African malaria falls mainly on the very young, and those who survive gradually develop an increasing immunity. This means that spectacular epidemic outbreaks are usually absent, but the disease kills many infants and young children, and contributes in a large measure to the vicious circle of disease and poverty.

Various malaria-control activities, especially the distribution of drugs for prevention and treatment of infection, are being carried out in urban and some rural areas, but the overall situation has not greatly improved in tropical Africa. On the other hand, one should point out that in northern and southern Africa malaria is either absent or definitely on the retreat, while its eradication has recently been accomplished in Mauritius and Reunion.

In other parts of the world, the situation varies between a slow but steady fall in the incidence of malaria and a virtual absence of any change. However, in several countries there is evidence of resurgence of malaria and this is causing much concern. Among these countries are Pakistan and Bangladesh, most parts of South-east Asia, Indonesia, Sri Lanka (Ceylon), and especially the states of Gujarat, Maharashtra, Madhya Pradesh and Rajasthan in India.

Since the malaria eradication programme of India is by far the largest in the world, its recent appraisal is of particular interest. During the period 1962–1976, the annual number of *reported* cases of malaria rose from 60 000 to over 5 million and the constant increase of the incidence is disquieting. In areas of the country inhabited by nearly 20 per cent of the population, the feasibility of eradication is doubtful under present administrative and economic conditions.

The present resurgence of malaria indicates how far we are from the conquest of this disease. It also emphasizes the role of malaria as one of the many factors at the core of the great issue of socio-economic development of tropical countries.

There is no denying that, in spite of the great achievements of the global programme, a large reservoir of endemic malaria remains over most of the tropics. The problems as seen in tropical Africa and Asia explain why the eradication of malaria from the whole of those continents is now considered unlikely as long as basic health services are qualitatively and quantitatively inadequate.

One of the consequences is the increasing concern with malaria as one of the tropical diseases now frequently seen in Europe, the USA, and other parts of the temperate world. The constantly rising speed and volume of international travel and the lure of exotic holidays at a moderate cost have created new conditions for massive importation of communicable disease into countries where these infections were unknown or from which they had gradually disappeared with the advance of public health. This is the appropriate place to mention the steady increase of imported malaria in Europe, North America and Japan. In Europe alone, where indigenous malaria has disappeared, the number of cases of imported malaria rose from 840 in 1967 to 2400 in 1976. It will be well over 3000 in 1977, with the highest figures in the UK, where in 1977 there were over 1500 cases and in 1978 nearly 2000. Malaria transmitted by blood transfusion is usually of imported origin and may have special features.

The main obstacles to the success of malaria control, let alone that of malaria eradication, are of administrative and operational nature. They range from shortages of trained manpower to inadequate Government support, premature integration of malaria eradication activities into general health services and various logistic difficulties of procurement of insecticides, drugs and transport.

Apart from these general problems, there are some of a more specifically technical nature. Among these one must mention resistance of anopheline vectors to insecticides and exophily of some *Anopheles* vectors. The use of alternative insecticides means greatly increased operational costs. Of special interest is a series of factors related to human ecology that interfere with antimalaria activities. Inaccessibility of some localities, the custom of replastering of houses for religious feasts or family events, reluctance of inhabitants (especially in traditional Moslem and other communities) to have their houses sprayed, and nomadic population movements are all of some importance. Urban malaria is a new phenomenon related to the rapid increase of urban populations, especially in India and Pakistan. Thus Karachi's population rose from 2 million in 1961 to 4 million in 1973; Lahore showed an increase from 1·3 million in 1961 to 2·2 million in 1972. Rapid extension of these two urban areas combined with digging innumerable foundations and borrow pits for poorly constructed houses led to the creation of many breeding places for local vectors and this was followed by an epidemic of malaria in Karachi with 600 000 cases in 1967. In Pakistan alone, the problem of urban malaria, due in part to administrative failures, involves a population of 10 million in nine major cities and more than 50 smaller towns. Realistic assessment of the difficulties that have stopped the striking advance of global malaria eradication recognizes the importance of administrative, socio-economic, financial, and political difficulties. These affect the problem of improving health in developing countries with low financial means, inadequate basic health services and shortages of trained manpower.

The relationship between malaria and socio-economic development has two aspects. Socio-economic advance may be largely responsible for the decrease if not disappearance of malaria; this has happened in most European countries. On the other hand, endemic malaria may delay economic and social development if the population bears a heavy burden of disease, an important factor in maintaining poverty and ignorance. It has been shown that in Central and South America the eradication of malaria was successful where the gross national income (GNI) was higher than US $500 per head of population; on the other hand the programme was a failure in seven countries with GNI lower than that figure. The national resources available for antimalaria programmes vary considerably from country to country, not always in relation to the total annual health budget. The weighted average for the latter in 25 countries of tropical Africa was US $1·20 *per capita* and this is rarely more than 2 per cent and at the most 5 per cent of the total annual budget. Out of this the funds allocated for specific antimalaria measures vary between 5 and 10 per cent of the annual health budget. Thus the appropriation for malaria control in Africa is well below the cost of minimal antimalaria control measures which were calculated in 1973 as US $0·35 per head per year.

A re-examination of the global strategy of malaria eradication was recommended by the 20th and 21st World Health Assemblies. Special studies on the socio-economic impact of malaria, the relationship of malaria eradication programmes to national health planning, and the technical or other aspects of malaria eradication activities have been carried out during the past few years and their results were presented to the 22nd World Health Assembly in 1969. The main conclusions of this report stress that malaria eradication should remain the final goal; a long-term investment because of its overall impact on health and its socio-economic benefits. Wherever malaria eradication programmes have good prospects, they should be pursued with vigour towards their defined goal. In countries where eradication does not appear to be feasible because of the inadequacy of financial resources, manpower requirements, or basic health services, malaria control operations may form a transitional stage towards the future launching of an eradication programme.

Within the general agreement on the urgency of better malaria control, three needs emerge: the improvement of basic health services, research into control techniques, and a reduction in the birth rate to balance the reduction in the death rate.

The expansion of health services is limited by the supply of trained manpower, especially in rural areas, where the needs are immense. It is here that the role of medical auxiliaries is of growing importance and much more must be done to increase their numbers as well as their skills and responsibilities. Our technical means of controlling, let alone eradicating, malaria in many endemic areas of the world are inadequate. A concentrated research effort may find new ways to attack the malaria parasite and its vector. Fields in which research is felt to be particularly important include the improvement of immunological surveillance techniques, study of the behaviour of mosquito vectors and their resistance to insecticides, better and more acceptable insecticides, and the development of new antimalarial drugs. Much has been said and written about the possibility of a prospective malaria vaccine, but the present experimental results, however encouraging, show the practical difficulties of this method. It seems that synthetic antimalarial drugs will be our most reliable weapon for many years. Nevertheless, research in the feasibility of malaria vaccine should be stimulated and supported.

On a world scale, the health gains of malaria eradication are immense; this can be judged from the fact that the 1950 annual malaria morbidity rate of about 250 million has now declined to about 100 million clinical cases. Moreover it has been shown that even in areas where malaria eradication was not successful, the mortality rate due to malaria and other vector-borne diseases has decreased quite spectacularly, on the average by 20 per cent. The corresponding global malaria mortality rate has decreased from 2·5 million to less than 1 million per annum. Over the past decade the probable reduction of mortality attributed directly to malaria amounted to some 50 million. This should be seen in the proper perspective of the general demographic trend as the world population increased during that period by about 600 million.

The impact of any large-scale control of an endemic disease is bound to lower the amount of sickness and death and thus increase the population pressure wherever a high reproductive potential exists. If the ideal aim of community medicine is to keep an ecological balance between human society and its environment, the drastic reduction of sickness and death should be counter-balanced by a corresponding reduction of the birth rate. Deliberate limitation of a family is a policy alien to most of the developing countries, especially those where the fearful mortality rates for infants and children indicate the burden of sickness carried by the young and are closely related to socio-economic conditions. A family needs to feel certain of survival before it gives some thought to limiting its size. Only when the protection of the health of the mother and child removes the instinctive fear of premature death will restrictive measures on procreation be adopted.

In considering the relationship of the population to the available resources, it would be unwise to think only of food production as the most serious potential shortage. The size of the population must be related also to the availability of social services, investment policy, industrial development, conservation of the natural environment and the resources of the land.

The pursuit of a well defined campaign against one specific disease may often provide an effective lever for economic progress if it lifts from the community a heavy burden of sickness. But this should be regarded as part of the general process of orderly growth of national health determined by existing priorities.

Today's problems of malaria control, let alone those of eradication, are part of the unsolved dilemma of the developing world. The current economic upheavals, which are a result of the energy crisis, may aggravate the situation, but wealthier countries must fully realize the future danger of a divided world and accept the obligation of providing adequate technical and financial assistance to bridge the present gulfs.

ECOLOGICAL FACTORS IN GASTROENTERITIS

M. G. M. ROWLAND

Medical Research Council Dunn Nutrition Unit,
Milton Road, Cambridge

and R. A. E. BARRELL

Public Health Laboratory, Withington Hospital,
Manchester

Introduction

ACUTE gastroenteritis is the clinical syndrome of diarrhoea and/or vomiting of acute onset, often accompanied by fever and constitutional disturbance, which is of infective origin and is not secondary to some primary disease process outside the alimentary tract (Walker-Smith, 1975).

Gastroenteritis is largely a disease of developing countries and of young children, about 80 per cent of cases occurring in children under the age of 2 years (Ransome-Kuti, 1976). In 1975 it was estimated that there were 500 million episodes of diarrhoea in children in Asia, Africa and Latin America, resulting in between 5 and 18 million deaths (Rohde and Northrup, 1976).

Aetiological agents in young children with diarrhoea are usually detected by stool examination. Bacterial pathogens may be found in from 5 to 60 per cent—an average figure of 35 per cent has been quoted (Cramblett, Azimi and Haynes, 1971). These organisms include *Shigellae*, *Salmonellae*, diarrhoeagenic *Escherichia coli* and *Vibrio cholerae*. More recently, rotaviruses and other viruses have been detected by electron microscopy of faeces (Middleton,

Szymanski and Petrie, 1977), and it has been realized that bacteria may be found in the upper gut which cause disease by virtue of their situation as well as their nature (Dammin, 1965).

Whatever the causal organisms, transmission is generally via the faeco–oral route — in other words, faecally contaminated material is transferred from one individual, or indeed animal, via water, food or fomite and is swallowed by the next victim. This group of diseases has been subdivided by Bradley who introduced and then updated the concept of a classification of water-related disease (Bradley, 1974) including the categories *water-borne* — classical cholera and typhoid have been quoted as examples in which contamination of water supplies is the prime cause — and *water-washed* — such as bacillary dysentery (shigellosis) where person-to-person contact and hygiene appear more important (van Zijl, 1966). The relevant section of the classification is shown in Table 1. Recently, however, the relationship has appeared much less clear-cut, as shown by experiences with cholera in Bangladesh (Curlin, Aziz and Khan, 1977) and with typhoid in Lesotho (Feachem *et al.*, 1978).

The main causal agents of conventional gastroenteritis are *Shigellae*, *Salmonellae*, diarrhoeagenic *E. coli* and *rotaviruses*. *Shigellosis (bacillary dysentery)* occurs worldwide and the incidence remains high although there has been an interesting change in the distribution of the specific organisms. Flexner and Shiga dysentery, often severe infections, predominate in the tropics, but in the more developed countries have been largely replaced by the milder Sonne dysentery (Christie, 1969; Fraser, Thornsberry and Feldman, 1972). It has been suggested that this is because the infectious dose of the types of organism that produce the more severe forms of the disease is higher than that of the less pathogenic organisms.

TABLE 1. Classification of infective diseases in relation to water supplies (from Bradley, 1974).

Category	Examples	Relevant water improvements
I Water-borne infections		
(a) Classical	Typhoid, cholera	Microbiological sterility
(b) Non-classical	Infective hepatitis	Microbiological improvement
II Water-washed infections		
(a) Skin and eyes	Scabies, trachoma	Greater volume available
(b) Diarrhoeal diseases	Bacillary dysentery	Greater volume available

Shigellosis affects all ages and the causative organisms are among the more frequently isolated bacteria in childhood diarrhoea (Abraham *et al.*, 1978; Gordon *et al.*, 1962). It is generally agreed that shigellosis is associated mainly with poverty, overcrowding and poor hygiene. It is spread by person-to-person contact, food, fomites and flies. It is classified as "water-washed" and this is justified by numerous studies which show that the incidence is inversely related to the availability of clean water for general use and drinking (Gordon *et al.*, 1962; Hollister *et al.*, 1955; van Zijl, 1966). The disease is less common during very hot dry months — it has been claimed that sunshine dries up the exposed faeces and kills fly maggots. The organism is shed by cases, by convalescents for up to 2 months or more, and by chronic carriers; so sanitation is clearly important.

Salmonellosis presents as a spectrum of febrile and gastrointestinal diseases. Apart from enteric fever and classical food poisoning, *Salmonellae* may be isolated in outbreaks of childhood diarrhoea or in the course of an illness which appears to be a gastroenteritis. Animal hosts such as poultry (Hobbs, 1961) and cattle (Moore, De la Cruz and Vargas Mendez, 1965) may be important as reservoirs of infection as well as man and this is probably spread via food and water. On the whole, however, *Salmonella* gastroenteritis appears surprisingly infrequently (Gordon *et al.*, 1962).

Diarrhoeagenic *E. coli* are mainly of importance in infancy (Cramblett *et al.*, 1971) in developed countries where they are particularly responsible for outbreaks of infection in baby nurseries. They may also cause travellers' diarrhoea (Gorbach *et al.*, 1975). They are relatively more common in childhood diarrhoeas in third world countries, probably because a relatively high dose is required to produce infection (Gangarosa, 1978).

These pathogens fall into three broad groups (Rowe, Gross and Scotland, 1976; Sack, 1976):

(*a*) enteropathogenic *E. coli*, identified by serotypes that are known to be associated with diarrhoeal epidemics;

(*b*) enterotoxigenic organisms, in which it is possible to demonstrate virulence by toxin production;

(*c*) enteroinvasive *E. coli*.

Food and water hygiene is probably more important in transmission than person-to-person contact, but an important host factor applies particularly in poor communities — breast-fed children seem to be much less susceptible to infection than artificially fed children, possibly because of the composition of their normal gut flora and perhaps also because of specific protective factors in breast milk (Hanson, 1976).

A major advance in our understanding of the aetiology of gastroenteritis has been the discovery in this decade of *rotaviruses* which have now been demonstrated worldwide, mainly in cases of childhood diarrhoea (*British Medical Journal*, 1975). Isolation rates of up to 85 per cent have been documented in some communities at certain times of the year (Bryden *et al.*, 1975). Cutting (1978) has recently reviewed the seasonal timing of these outbreaks, which appear to occur mainly in the cold or winter season in temperate zones, although rainfall may be more important in some areas of the tropics. Human milk contains antiviral activity, so breast feeding may protect against symptomatic disease in human infants (Thouless, Bryden and Flewett, 1978) — certainly colostrum is a vital protective factor in some animals such as the calf (Woode, Jones and Bridger, 1975).

The last 50 years have seen a change in the pattern of diarrhoeas in the developed countries. The phenomena of summer diarrhoea thought to be of bacterial origin (e.g., *Salmonella*) has been largely replaced in importance by winter diarrhoea of viral origin (Ramos-Alvarez and Sabin, 1958). We do not know the reason for this. Rotavirus diarrhoea contributes significantly to the morbidity and mortality of gastroenteritis throughout the world, including some cases in adults (Von Bonsdorff *et al.*, 1976), but the illness it produces is self-limiting and amenable to medical treatment in the form of fluid and electrolyte therapy. Furthermore, there is hope that a vaccine may be developed against it, though it now seems that a polyvalent preparation may be required (Zissis and Lambert, 1978).

Despite this prosepct, there still remains the most complex and intractable of all the forms of gastroenteritis, that of the weanling diarrhoea syndrome. This term was coined by Gordon, Chitkara and Wyon (1963) to describe the particularly high and disastrous prevalence of diarrhoea observed in young Guatemalan children from about 6 to 18 or 24 months of age during the period when food is introduced to supplement the mothers' breast milk. This disease exacts a heavy toll in terms of growth, morbidity and mortality and is a major problem throughout the developing world.

The Keneba Project

Since 1974, the Medical Research Council (MRC) Dunn Nutrition Unit has carried out a detailed epidemiological study of malnutrition or growth failure in young children in The Gambia, West Africa. It would be inappropriate to discuss growth and dietary patterns in detail in this paper, but it should be mentioned that it was demonstrated that in this community a major cause of morbidity and failure to thrive is diarrhoeal illness or gastroenteritis (Rowland, Cole and Whitehead, 1977). The main brunt of the illness is borne by children in late infancy and the second year of life and is an example of the weanling diarrhoea syndrome. Two facts will suffice to show how severe the problem is. First, during certain seasons children in the above age group have diarrhoea on average for 1 week in every month. Secondly, in the first five years, one half of these children die (McGregor, 1976) and many of these deaths are almost certainly linked with malnutrition and gastroenteritis.

Because of this devastating picture of diarrhoeal disease, we endeavoured to discover its aetiology. Like so many other workers, we found very little to explain it when we examined stools. Bacteria such as *Shigellae, Salmonellae* and pathogenic *E. coli* were isolated in only about 6 per cent of cases and *rotaviruses* were absent at the time of the survey. A remarkable finding, however, was that one half of the children in this vulnerable age group had an abnormal distribution of the gut flora; i.e., excessively high bacterial counts in the jejunum. An even higher proportion had biochemical evidence strongly suggestive of disturbed gut function (Rowland and McCollum, 1977). These findings are summarized in Table 2. Clearly, if such a situation is to be remedied or prevented, it is necessary to understand the contributing ecological factors.

TABLE 2. Summary of aetiological findings in weanling diarrhoea in Keneba (from Rowland and McCollum, 1977).

Stool pathogen isolation	5%
Rotavirus isolation	nil
Giardia lamblia	16%
Jejunal bacteria $\geq 10^5$/ml	52%
Disturbed bile salt metabolism	53–80%

In this field there is little difference between disease in the country and in the town, probably because many of the sprawling shantytown suburbs in developing countries exhibit the same lack of facilities and technology as rural areas. Moreover, gastroenteritis is

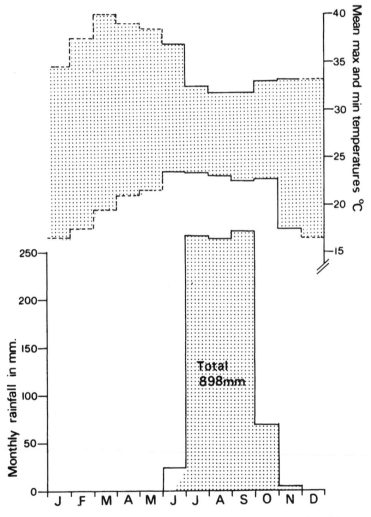

FIG. 1. Keneba meteorological data 1974–77, monthly means of rainfall, mean maximum and mean minimum temperature. - - - - - available data less than 3 years.

TABLE 3. Simplified Keneba annual events calendar.

Month	Weather	Activity	Food availability	Other
Dec Jan Feb	Dry and largely cool	Tail end of harvest Trade	All food good	Easiest time of year
March April	Increasingly hot	Building (men) Little burning off and clearing	Dwindling stocks, some food bought	Cash in hand, little illness
May June	Start of rains to	Intensive clearing and planting	Poor stocks and cash shortage	Some co-op loans and food aid
July Aug	peak period			Peak of child morbidity
Sept Oct Nov	Fall off and cessation of rains	Weeding, crop guarding. harvesting	Improving with harvesting of early crops (*Zea* and *Digitaria*)	and mortality

particularly a problem of developing countries, in which in 1970, 72 per cent of the population lived in rural areas (World Health Organization, 1973).

Keneba village, the site of the MRC study, has a population of about 1000 and lies in the sub-Sahel. The pattern of life in this subsistence farming community is largely controlled by the climate. The rains are strictly monomodal, between 20 and 40 in. falling from June to October each year; and, as shown in Fig. 1, the hottest time of the year precedes the rains in March to May. Humidity is high throughout the rainy period and, in fact, starts to rise before the rains. Not surprisingly, activities can be very much categorized by the season of the year, as shown in the events calendar (Table 3).

Results

To determine the ecological factors here, let us first consider the seasonal variation of gastroenteritis. Over the last four years, there has been a striking relationship with the rains. The picture for 1977 is illustrated in Fig. 2. In each year the increase in the prevalence of diarrhoea preceded the onset of the rains by about 4 to 6 weeks (being least striking in the 1977 data). This may be because the rise in humidity enhances the survival of pathogens, but there are other possibilities. There is a period of water shortage every year towards the end of the dry season before the new rains replenish the water table. The six wells which supply the village are only about 20 m deep and two at least may dry up during bad years. There is, therefore, a shortage of water. The fly population at this time was not studied, but experience elsewhere suggests that the numbers would not reach a peak until the rains were well established.

However, the main peak of diarrhoeal illness occurs unequivocally about the middle of the rains and it is natural to ask what happens to water purity during this period. Water from these wells is faecally polluted at all times and would be totally unacceptable in developed countries (Barrell and Rowland, 1979b). Within days of the onset of the first rains, the level of pollution rises 10- to 100-fold and this pattern is generally sustained throughout the rainy season, after which it gradually falls to its basic level.

The next question is how this might relate to the diarrhoeal pattern of the young child, who is not usually thought of as drinking much water. Surprisingly, in fact, in this area even young breast-fed infants

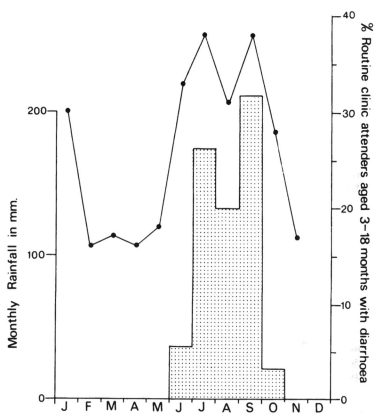

FIG. 2. Monthly rainfall ⬚ and monthly period prevalence of weanling diarrhoea ●———● in Keneba, 1977.

are given raw well water to drink from birth, though how much we do not yet know. It appears that on the whole the protection conferred by breast milk, which is universally consumed by the young infants of this village, defends them against these early and possibly minor insults. But despite continued breast-feeding, the protective mechanism starts to fail at around 6 months and diarrhoea becomes increasingly common. This could be due to declining host resistance, as growth impairment has already started at this age (Whitehead *et al.*, 1977). But at 6 months, malnutrition is not severe and is probably not the explanation. In fact, on a seasonal basis the incidence of diarrhoea reaches its peak at the time when nutritional status of children is optimal (Rowland, unpublished).

However, from 4 to 6 months of age, weaning foods in the form of traditional cereal gruels, often rice or millet flour cooked with water, are introduced in steadily increasing amounts. Although one might expect a cooked food to be safe, the mother is constrained by the fairly limited type of food which a young infant can consume. The food is rarely boiled properly as it becomes too glutinous for her baby to cope with.

In fact, *Bacillus cereus* (known to cause outbreaks of food poisoning in the UK when reheated rice dishes are served up, for instance in Chinese restaurants) is an ubiquitous organism in this cereal-producing community. The water with which the cereal flour is mixed contains faecal organisms and more faecal coliforms are introduced later in the course of preparation. The levels of this contamination at any given time after cooking are definitely higher during the rains (Barrell and Rowland, 1979a) than in the dry season.

The time that elapses after food is cooked and before it is eaten is related to an important ecological factor, namely the work burden of the mothers. The womenfolk participate fully in the very intensive seasonal farming activities. The fields are cleared before the rains and planted and weeded in the first half of the rains and during these periods the women may spend 10 to 12 hours away from home. Pregnancy or the presence of a young child are no grounds for absence, although until their infant reaches 3 months, women rarely undertake such heavy labouring duties. After this, however, children are either taken to the fields by their mothers or, increasingly as they get older, they are left at home in the care of young 'nursemaids', often between 7 and 10 years old. In this situation, instead of producing a fresh cooked meal for each sitting, mothers tend to prepare food in bulk at the start of the day and the child dips into this throughout the mother's absence. The scope for bacterial overgrowth and super-added contamination is obvious and the end result is illustrated in Table 4. Thus towards the end of the day during the wet season, infants are regularly consuming food which is dangerous to health.

This then is the background to the annual rainy season epidemic of weanling diarrhoea which appears to be a bacterial phenomenon consequent upon bacterial overgrowth of the upper gut.

TABLE 4. The percentages of Gambian weaning food samples containing unacceptable levels of pathogens as defined by the International Commission on Microbiological Specifications for Foods, 1974 (after Barrell and Rowland, 1979a).

Time elapsed after cooking, (h)	Percentage unacceptable during	
	Rains (June–Nov)	Dry (Dec–May)
0–1	35	7
1–2	53	31
4–6	58	46
8	96	71

There do, however, appear to be minor peaks occurring in the middle of the dry season when the weather is still cool. A typical secondary peak in January 1977 is shown in Fig. 1. We can only speculate on the nature of these at present, but we do know that rotavirus, absent from the rainy season study, is nevertheless a common infecting organism in the children, as shown by a retrospective sero-survey (unpublished results) and these small peaks may be caused by rotavirus epidemics. These appear to be of considerably less importance to the health of the children than the diarrhoea of the wet season and the attacks of disease are short-lived.

Discussion

The ecological factors bearing on the nature and spread of gastroenteritis fall into three broad categories: the physical environment, the social environment and host factors.

In Keneba, humidity, rainfall, the availability of water, water pollution and the virtual absence of sanitation facilities appear to be the main components of the first group. Maternal deprivation seems to be a major social problem. The poor diet and nutritional status of the mothers impairs lactation, so supplementary infant feeding is needed as early as the fourth month of age (Whitehead et al., 1978). The mothers lack knowledge and facilities for sterilizing feeds and for storing clean water, and the standards of child care and infant feeding are poor because of the exorbitant seasonal demands made upon them to work in the field; as a result, young children are repeatedly fed highly contaminated, poorly nutritious diets. The practice of breast-feeding well into the second year of life is a valuable support to children in such unhygienic surroundings, but the protection it gives declines or disappears in the second half of infancy. This probably results both because increasing quantities of contaminated material are consumed and because immunity is waning.

It is unlikely that any single input can effect a radical improvement in such a situation — a fairly general improvement in living standards appears vital. Nevertheless, we should have some target in mind and one such is to improve environmental hygiene and sanitation. The fundamental need for this is supported by the differences between the clinical features of gastroenteritis and its aetiology in industrialized and in third world countries. A World Health Organization report (1973) has suggested that 86 per cent of the rural population of developing countries, amounting to over 1 billion people, lack a plentiful supply of clean water. The logistic problem of rectifying this is enormous, as Feachem (1975) has pointed out. But we should not forget that in this country 50 years ago the state of environmental hygiene and its attendant gastroenteritis resembled that seen in many developing countries today (Drasar, Tomkins and Feachem, 1978). Despite encouraging results in treating gastroenteritis with fluid and electrolytes, the benefits are not as marked in the very young as in older children (Hirschhorn, 1977; Rowland and Cole, 1980). An antiviral vaccine, when developed, may well prove to have similar limitations. The solution must be to improve preventive public health measures.

The value of water improvement schemes is uncertain. Experience in Bangladesh has shown that introducing tube wells to supply clean potable drinking water to villages failed completely to reduce the incidence of El Tor cholera in the population (Sommer and Woodward, 1972). The reason for this is not clearly understood (Briscoe, 1977) but is almost certainly related to the fact that large amounts of grossly contaminated water continued to be used for all other purposes, including cooking and bathing. The lack of demonstrable benefit in Lesotho water improvement schemes (Feachem et al., 1978) is equally unsatisfactory.

On balance it seems likely that to have a significant effect on the incidence of disease, water improvements must be comprehensive: that the supply of clean water should be so accessible and generous that it completely supplants the use of unprotected supplies. At present this seems impossible in Keneba — such a scheme would not be practical because it could not be maintained and would be too expensive. But it should be practicable and affordable in urban communities. Gastroenteritis is not an urban disease unless the population there lacks facilities and continues to live in squalor. The current worldwide drift to the towns is often lamented, but it could be exploited to ensure that more and more people, even in poor third world countries, enjoy a water supply and sanitation of a basic standard and so enjoy also a reduction in one of the major diseases of young children, gastroenteritis.

Acknowledgement

The authors thank Dr. D. A. J. Tyrrell of the Clinical Research Centre, Harrow, for very considerable help and advice in the preparation of this manuscript.

References

ABRAHAM, A. A., CAHILL, K. M., DAVIES, J., KAWAGUCHI, T., MILLER, L. F., NORTHWAY, J. D. and DAMMIN, G. J. (1978) Studies on Infantile Diarrhoea in Cairo, Egypt. *Journal of Tropical Pediatrics and Environmental Child Health*, **24**, 187–194.

BARRELL, R. A. E. and ROWLAND, M. G. M. (1979 a), Infant foods as a potential source of diarrhoeal illness in rural West Africa. *Transactions of the Royal Society of Tropical Medicine and Hygiene*, **73**, 85–90.

BARRELL, R. A. E. and ROWLAND, M. G. M. (1979 b) The relationship between rainfall and well water pollution in a West African (Gambian) village. *Journal of Hygiene, Cambridge*. **83**, 143 150.

BRADLEY, D. J. (1974) Water supplies: the consequence of change. In *Human Rights in Health*, Ciba Foundation Symposium 23, p. 81. Amsterdam: Elsevier/Excerpta Medica/North Holland.

BRISCOE, J. (1977) The role of water supply in improving health in poor countries (with special reference to Bangladesh). *Scientific Report No. 6, Cholera Research Laboratory*, p. 3 Dacca: Bangladesh.

BRITISH MEDICAL JOURNAL EDITORIAL (1975) Virus of infantile gastroenteritis. *British Medical Journal*, iii, 555–556.

BRYDEN, A. S., DAVIES, A. A., HADLEY, R. E., FLEWETT, T. H., MORRIS, C. A. and OLIVER, P. (1975) Rotavirus in the West Midlands during 1974. *Lancet*, ii, 241–243.

CHRISTIE, A. B. (1969) Bacillary dysentery. In *Diseases of the Digestive System*, p. 190. London: British Medical Association.

CRAMBLETT, H. G., AZIMI, P. and HAYNES, R. E. (1971) The etiology of infectious diarrhea in infancy, with special reference to enteropathogenic E. coli. *Annals of the New York Academy of Sciences*, **176**, 80–92.

CURLIN, G. T., AZIZ, K. M. A. and KHAN, M. R. (1977) The Influence of Drinking Tube well Water on Diarrhoea Rates in Matlab Thana, Bangladesh. *Working Paper No. 1, Cholera Research Laboratory*, p. 18. Dacca, Bangladesh.

CUTTING, W. A. M. (1978) Seasonal variations in rotavirus infection and diarrhoea in childhood. In paper presented at a Conference on *Seasonal Dimensions to Rural Poverty*, held at the Institute of Development Studies, University of Sussex, 3–6 July, p. 8.

DAMMIN, G. J. (1965) Pathogenesis of acute clinical diarrhoeal disease. *Federation Proceedings*, **24**, 35–38.

DRASAR, B. S., TOMKINS, A. M. and FEACHEM, R. G. (1978) Seasonal aspects of diarrhoeal disease. In paper presented at a Conference on *Seasonal Dimensions to Rural Poverty* held at the Institute of Development Studies, University of Sussex, 3–6 July, p. 34.

FEACHEM, R. G. (1975) Water Supplies for low-Income Communities in Developing Countries. *Journal of the Environmental Engineering Division, ASCE*, **101**, 687–702.

FEACHEM, R. G., BURNS, E., CAIRNCROSS, A. M., CRONIN, A., CROSS, P., CURTIS, D., KHAN, M. K., LAMB, D. and SOUTHALL, H. A. (1978) Water Supplies and Disease in Lesotho. In *Water, Health and Development*, p. 144. London: Trimed Books Ltd.

FRASER, D. W., THORNSBERRY, C. and FELDMAN, R. A. (1972) Shigellosis in the United States, 1970. *Journal of Infectious Diseases*, **125**, 441–446.

GANGAROSA, E. J. (1978) Epidemiology of *Escherichia coli* in the United States. *Journal of Infectious Diseases*, **137**, 634–638.

GORBACH, S. L., KEAN, B. H., EVANS, D. G., EVANS, D. J. and BESSUDO, D. (1975) Travelers' diarrhea and toxigenic *Escherichia coli*. *New England Journal of Medicine*, **292**, 933–936.

GORDON, J. E., PIERCE, V., ASCOLI, W. and SCRIMSHAW, N. S. (1962) Studies of diarrheal disease in Central America. II. Community prevalence of *Shigella* and *Salmonella* infections in childhood populations of Guatemala. *American Journal of Tropical Medicine and Hygiene*, **11**, 389–394.

GORDON, J. E., CHITKARA, I. D. and WYON, J. B. (1963) Weanling diarrhea. *American Journal of Medical Science*, **245**, 345–377.

HANSON, L. Å. (1976) *Esch. coli* infections in childhood. *Archives of Disease in Childhood*, **51**, 737–743.

HIRSCHHORN, N. (1977) A positive effect on the nutrition of Philippine children of an oral glucose-electrolyte solution given at home for the treatment of diarrhoea. *Bulletin of the World Health Organization*, **55**, 87–94.

HOBBS, B. C. (1961) Public health significance of *Salmonella* carriers in livestock and birds. *Journal of Applied Bacteriology*, **24**, 340–352.

HOLLISTER, A. C., BECK, M. D., GITTELSOHN, A. M. and HEMPHILL, E. C. (1955) Influence of Water Availability on *Shigella* Prevalence in Children of Farm Labor Families. *American Journal of Public Health*, **45**, 354–362.

INTERNATIONAL COMMISSION ON MICROBIOLOGICAL SPECIFICATIONS FOR FOODS OF THE INTERNATIONAL ASSOCIATION OF MICROBIOLOGICAL SOCIETIES (1974) *Microorganisms in Foods*, Vol. 2. Toronto: University of Toronto Press.

MCGREGOR, I. A. (1976) Health and communicable disease in a rural African environment. *Oikos*, **27**, 180–192.

MIDDLETON, P. J., SZYMANSKI, M. T. and PETRIE, M. (1977) Viruses Associated with Acute Gastroenteritis in Young Children. *American Journal of Diseases in Childhood*, **131**, 733–737.

MOORE, H. A., DE LA CRUZ, E. and VARGAS MENDEZ, O. (1965) Diarrheal disease studies in Costa Rica. IV. The influence of sanitation upon the prevalence of intestinal infection and diarrheal disease. *American Journal of Epidemiology*, **82**, 162–184.

RAMOS-ALVAREZ, M. and SABIN, A. B. (1958) Enteropathogenic viruses and bacteria. Role in summer diarrheal diseases of infancy and early childhood. *Journal of the American Medical Association*, 167, 147–156.

RANSOME-KUTI, O. (1976) Gastroenteritis in infants. In *Principles of Medicine in Africa*, ed. PARRY, E. H. O. p. 169. Oxford: Oxford University Press.

ROHDE, J. E. and NORTHRUP, R. S. (1976) Taking science where the diarrhoea is. In *Acute Diarrhoea in Childhood*, Ciba Foundation Symposium 42, ed. ELLIOTT, K., p. 339. Amsterdam: Elsevier/Excerpta Medica/North Holland.

ROWE, B., GROSS, R. J. and SCOTLAND, S. M. (1976) Serotyping of *E. coli. Lancet*, ii, 37–38.

ROWLAND, M. G. M., COLE, T. J. and WHITEHEAD, R. G. (1977) A quantitative study into the role of infection in determining nutritional status in Gambian village children. *British Journal of Nutrition*, 37, 441–450.

ROWLAND, M. G. M. and MCCOLLUM, J. P. K. (1977) Malnutrition and Gastroenteritis in The Gambia. *Transactions of the Royal Society of Tropical Medicine and Hygiene*, 71, 199 203.

ROWLAND, M. G. M. and COLE, T. J. (1980) The effect of early glucose-electrolyte therapy on diarrhoea and growth in rural Gambian village children, *Journal of Tropical Pediatrics and Environmental Child Health*, 26 (in the press).

SACK, R. B. (1976) Serotyping of *E. coli, Lancet*, i, 1132.

SOMMER, A. and WOODWARD, W. (1972) The influence of protected water supplies on the spread of classical/Inaba and El Tor/Ogawa cholera in rural East Bengal. *Lancet*, ii, 985–987.

THOULESS, M. E., BRYDEN, A. S. and FLEWETT, T. H. (1978) Rotavirus neutralization by human milk. *British Medical Journal*, ii, 1390.

WALKER-SMITH, J. (1975) Gastroenteritis, In *Diseases of the Small Intestine in Childhood*, 1st edn., p. 110. London: Pitman Medical.

WHITEHEAD, R. G., COWARD, W. A., LUNN, P. G. and RUTISHAUSER, I. H. E. (1977) A comparison of the pathogenesis of protein-energy malnutrition in Uganda and The Gambia. *Transactions of the Royal Society of Tropical Medicine and Hygiene*, 71, 189–195.

WHITEHEAD, R. G., ROWLAND, M. G. M., HUTTON, M. A., PRENTICE, A. M., MÜLLER, E. and PAUL, A. A. (1978) Factors influencing lactation performance in rural Gambian mothers. *Lancet*, ii, 178–181.

WOODE, G. N., JONES, J. and BRIDGER, J. C. (1975) Levels of colostral antibodies against neonatal calf diarrhoea virus. *Veterinary Record*, 97, 148–149.

WORLD HEALTH ORGANIZATION (1973) *World Health Statistics Report*, 26, No. 11.

VAN ZUL, W. J. (1966) Studies on Diarrhoeal Diseases in Seven Countries by the WHO Diarrhoeal Diseases Advisory Team. *Bulletin of the World Health Organization*, 35, 249–261.

VON BONSDORFF, C.-H., HOVI, T., MÅKELÅ, P., HOVI, L. and TEVALVOTO-AARNIO, M. (1976) Rotavirus associated with acute gastroenteritis in adults. *Lancet*, ii, 423.

ZISSIS, G. and LAMBERT, J. P. (1978) Different serotypes of human rotavirus. *Lancet*, i, 38–39.

NUTRITION AND INFECTIOUS DISEASE

D. C. MORLEY

Tropical Paediatrics Unit, Institute of Child Health, London

THE worldwide distribution of childhood malnutrition and infection is closely associated with poverty and lack of justice in meeting basic human needs. No other criterion of the quality of life shows so directly the level of need in a society or in the world community. In the past, improvement in child health and nutrition has had to wait for general socio-economic development. We now have an additional possibility of developing specific programmes which will help the less privileged children of our world escape from this vicious cycle produced by the interaction of nutrition and infection.

The care of diseases such as typhoid and tuberculosis was revolutionized when it was found that maintaining nutritional status was important, and that any kind of fever caused massive protein loss. Measles is perhaps the disease which illustrates the complexity of the interaction better than any other. It is recognized that measles precipitates malnutrition, and epidemics of kwashiorkor may follow epidemics of measles (Mata, Urrutia and Lechtig, 1971). The severe measles seen in Africa and in other areas where malnutrition exists may have a mortality around 400 times as great as measles in a well nourished community. Lastly, the malnourished child with measles probably remains infective far longer than a well nourished child. As a result, opportunities of infection are much higher and measles in most developing countries is a disease of the first three years of life, a period when the child is particularly at nutritional risk.

In this paper an attempt will be made to identify possible priorities if this massive problem of interaction between nutrition and infection which leads to so much more morbidity and mortality is to be tackled.

Size of the Problem

In our world today at least three out of four children live in the so-called developing countries (Fig. 1). Not only are there a large number of children, but as this figure shows, in the decade 1970 to 1980 the number of children in the developing countries increased by 300 million, i.e., the population of children in these countries was increased by the number of children living in Europe and North America.

For the Year of the Child, 1979, UNICEF estimated that there were 350 million children who live without even the minimum of health and educational services. Probably over 97 per cent of all deaths in children under 5 occur in developing countries. Common infections precipitate malnutrition which reduces resistance. Poor nutrition encourages more severe infection and again there is increased nutritional deficit. So often this sequence moves rapidly and the patient dies even though neither malnutrition nor infection by themselves would have caused death. This interaction is responsible for up to one half of the 45 million unnecessary child deaths under 5 each year in developing countries.

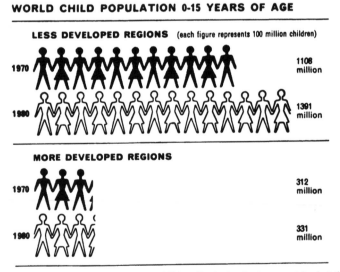

WORLD CHILD POPULATION 0-15 YEARS OF AGE

LESS DEVELOPED REGIONS (each figure represents 100 million children)

1970   1108 million

1980   1391 million

MORE DEVELOPED REGIONS

1970   312 million

1980   331 million

FIG. 1.   Not only do the majority of the children live in developing countries, but their number is increasing rapidly.

In these countries infections are concentrated in the early years of life and the second year is particularly dangerous. A comparison of the incidence of infections in the second year of life in the town of Newcastle upon Tyne in England and a rural area of Uganda is shown in Fig. 2. From this figure it will be seen that pneumonia is about ten times as common and diarrhoea six times as common in the African village child. Overall, the child is likely to have around five times as many episodes of illness, and between the ages of 6 months and 2 years will be off his food with some infection for 1 day in 3.

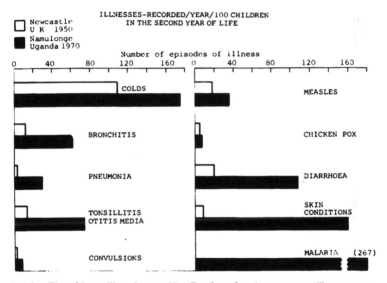

FIG. 2.   The African village 2-year old suffers from five times as many illnesses as an English child (Parkin, 1974).

Why are European Children Healthy?

The answer to this question is not as simple as it may seem. Antibiotics and immunization have only played a relatively small part, as the major decline in mortality in children occurred before either antibiotics or immunizations became widely available. In the past, much emphasis has been placed on clean water supplies, a cleaner environment and satisfactory sanitation. McKeown (1977) has recently questioned whether even more emphasis should not now be placed on improved nutrition. However, in his arguments to support nutrition, he hardly includes two illnesses, measles and diarrhoea, which are particularly significant, and if these are included, his arguments are that much stronger. European children now have better nutrition. This is not because of more and better protein, which probably plays a relatively small part. The important change has been that children in Europe over the last two centuries have had increasing access to foods with a concentrated energy content. In the developing world, where children are weaned on to paps and porridges of unrefined carbohydrate, the child, even if fed three meals a day, will have great difficulty in receiving sufficient energy. A study in East Africa showed that when children came off the breast in the second year of life, in spite of the mother giving them 60 per cent more staple, they were still deficient on energy. Breast milk is one of the ideal foods in terms of concentrated energy and the ease with which a child can take it.

We may speculate that improvement in the nutrition of children started in the 19th century with the introduction of steel milling of cereals and the removal of more and more dietary fibre from the childrens' diet. At the same time other foods, particularly dairy products and refined sugar, became more readily available, so that the mother had little difficulty in providing a high-energy diet. Unfortunately, this low-fibre and high-energy diet may now be one of the reasons for a constellation of diseases so common in Europe but unknown in the African village. Appendicitis and diverticulitis are almost certainly due to the depletion of dietary fibre, and depletion of this in European diets may be responsible in part for a number of other conditions as diverse as colonic cancer and ischaemic heart disease (Burkitt, 1975; Painter, 1975).

Priority Programmes to Influence the Interaction of Nutrition and Infection

When choosing the priority, various factors have to be considered; the four most important are community concern, prevalence, severity and manageability. Four possible priorities have been set out in Table 1 and these will be considered in turn. In this table a scale of + to + + + + is used and the result are multiplied to give a total score. This technique is meaningful to the author but the scores given and the methodology are open to many criticisms.

TABLE 1. Possible priorities to influence the interaction between nutrition and infection.

Programme	Community concern	Prevalence	Severity	Manageability	Score
Prevention of dehydration from episodes of diarrhoea	+ + +	+ + + +	+ + +	+ + + +	144
Increase energy intake	+ +	+ + + +	+ + +	+ +	48
Immunization	+ +	+ + +	+ + + +	+ +	48
Treatment of episodes of illness	+ + +	+ + + +	+ +	+	24

Prevention of dehydration in diarrhoea

My first priority would be to overcome and, where possible, prevent dehydration occurring. The weanling-aged child will have on average two episodes of diarrhoea every year and the malnourished child of this age, four. Repeated episodes of diarrhoea have been shown in The Gambia to carry the child into malnutrition. Almost all communities are concerned about diarrhoea and there is little doubt as to its severity, as in many countries it is the most important cause of death in small children. Reports from various areas around the world suggest that where oral rehydration is taught and practised satisfactorily at village level, severely dehydrated children are no longer frequently admitted to the hospital. A simple spoon, Fig. 3, described from Indonesia has proved so satisfactory that now a million are being produced (Hendrata, 1978).

Increased energy intake

The second priority is less obvious and is more likely to vary from community to community. Malnutrition and undernutrition is still not widely understood by communities and the majority still expect their children to be small and undergrown. However, it is highly prevalent and probably 80 per cent of children in most communities are undernourished at some stage and may show some degree of stunting. It is severe because of its effect on illness and also its

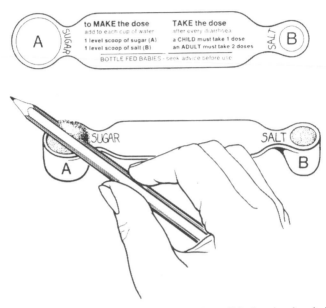

to MAKE the dose	TAKE the dose
add to each cup of water	after every diarrhoea
1 level scoop of sugar (A)	a CHILD must take 1 dose
1 level scoop of salt (B)	an ADULT must take 2 doses

BOTTLE FED BABIES - seek advice before use

Fig. 3. The simple spoon with the instructions that will be imprinted on it. If only rehydration can start with the first diarrhoeal stool, morbidity, malnutrition and mortality will be reduced.

potential in perhaps limiting the intellectual development of the child. Undernutrition is not easily manageable because the edible oils from which foods of high energy concentration can be produced are not always available in a village. Nor is the understanding of this requirement for concentrated high-energy foods, along with an adequate protein intake, appreciated by health workers and the community.

Immunization

While great emphasis is being placed on this, particularly with the expanded programme on immunization being undertaken by the World Health Organization, there is still a lack of understanding of its need at community level. Unfortunately, the natural history of common infections is still not a subject taught in the schools and as a priority in health education. Every child in our world is likely to suffer from measles unless vaccinated, and the majority will get whooping cough. Recently poliomyelitis, which has not been considered so severe, has been shown to leave flaccid paralysis in two to seven of every 1000 schoolchildren in studies in Ghana, Egypt and Burma. These illnesses, from which children can be protected, are the most severe infections from which most children suffer and yet with immunization the majority can be protected. Unfortunately, we do not yet have the logistics at village level to make this possible in the majority of countries.

Treatment of episodes of illness

Treatment is, of course, highly desired by the people and, as shown in Fig. 2, there is a high prevalence of communicable diseases, although many of them produce only minor illnesses. In a large proportion of these illnesses their management is particularly difficult because it calls for health workers who are accepted by the parents and who live within a kilometre of their home, if treatment is to be obtained.

Summary

The interaction of nutrition and infection is the major cause of the continuing high mortality among small children in developing countries. Of the many steps that may be taken to meet the situation, the management of dehydration has a high priority. After this, increasing the energy intake and immunization are likely to be the steps which will bring most benefit.

References

BURKITT, D. P. (1975) Appendicitis. In *Refined Carbohydrate Foods and Disease*, eds. BURKITT, D. P. and TROWELL, H. C., pp. 87–97. London: Academic Press.
HENDRATA, L. (1978) Spoons for making glucose–salt solution. *Lancet*, i, 612.
McKEOWN, T. (1977) *The Modern Rise of Population*. London: Edward Arnold.
MATA, L. J., URRUTIA, J. J. and LECHTIG, A. (1971) Infection and nutrition of children of a low socio-economic rural community. *American Journal of Clinical Nutrition*, 24, 249–259.
PAINTER, N. S. (1975) *Diverticular Disease of the Colon*, pp. 278–284. London: Heinemann.
PARKIN, J. M. (1974) A longitudinal study of village children in Uganda. In *The Child in the African Environment*, ed. OWOR, R. Nairobi: East African Literature Bureau.

MODELLING THE TRANSMISSION OF RABIES

P. ARMITAGE

Department of Biomathematics, University of Oxford

Introduction

RABIES is present throughout a large and increasing part of continental Europe, and the possibility of its introduction to the UK raises important questions of control strategy which we must keep under continual review. I want to talk about an aspect of epidemiology which particularly interests me as a statistician—the formation of quantitative models for the transmission of a disease. For some diseases, models have been developed and explored for many decades (Bailey, 1975; Cohen, 1977; Macdonald, 1973) and have helped to predict the effect on transmission of alternative control measures. In rabies, the history of modelling is much shorter, but it is interesting to consider the ways in which one might approach the task of modelling this disease, and to identify the biological information which is needed to enable useful results to emerge.

The nature of rabies

Rabies is a viral disease attacking the central nervous system, and is transmitted to man normally from the saliva of an infected animal—usually through a bite from an infected dog or cat. The disease in man is clinically appalling and almost invariably fatal, although not every bite from an infected animal leads to the clinical disease. Moreover, a human being can be protected by vaccination before a possible bite (if he or she is thought to be particularly at risk) or after a bite before symptoms occur. Similarly, domestic animals can be protected by systematic vaccination programmes.

In countries where rabies occurs there is normally a wildlife population among which the disease is endemic (or enzootic, to use the non-medical term). In Europe the main wildlife vector is the red fox. The problem of controlling the disease is therefore very different in countries with this permanently infected wildlife reservoir from that in countries like the UK in which wildlife is disease-free.

Rabies was widespread in Britain in the 19th century: rabid dogs were common and many human deaths occurred. Quarantine and the strict control of stray animals were introduced in 1897 and rabies had disappeared by 1903. There was a brief re-introduction to the dog population in 1919–1922, and there have been a few isolated incidents since then. Human rabies has been confined to a few people who acquired the infection abroad.

In Europe the disease has been established in the red fox population since the last war, and has affected some other species to a much lesser extent. The enzootic has gradually moved westwards and southwards. Denmark was cleared for many years by the establishment of a 'fox-free' zone along the border, but it has recently been re-invaded. Italy had its first recorded case of fox rabies in 1977. The rate of advance is irregular, but rates varying between about 10 and 80 km a year are reported, with an average of perhaps around 50 km a year. The front in France is quite close to Paris, although it seems recently to have slowed down and become less clearly defined, with isolated foci appearing at considerable distances from other reported cases.

Most European countries have, like the North American countries, accustomed themselves to the presence of rabies. Rigorous programmes of registration and vaccination of domestic pets, and the destruction of stray animals, are adopted, and the public becomes aware of the need for prophylactic measures after possible human exposure. Rabies is therefore not numerically an important disease of man in Europe, and the position is continually improving. Between 1972 and 1976 there were over 600 human deaths; during the last quarter of 1977 only one death was reported. Clearly, though, this public health control is achieved at the cost of a great deal of administrative effort and no-one can regard with equanimity the destruction, by rabies or by deliberate slaughter, of large numbers of animals, or the inevitable damage to our affectionate and tolerant relationship with wild animals. The world picture is much more disturbing. The incidence is unknown because of the gross under-reporting in developing countries, but one rough estimate is of 15 000 annual deaths in India alone (Schwabe, 1971).

The control policy in the UK is based in the first place on the preservation of effective quarantine. From time to time, perhaps increasingly often, breaches of quarantine regulations will occur. From any one rabid dog the chances of transmission to wildlife are probably small, but the control authorities will naturally be unwilling to take any appreciable risk. The policy will be to destroy wildlife, particularly the fox, within a limited radius. On the continent foxes are killed mainly by gassing, but in the UK poisoned bait is likely to be used.

The crucial question for the epidemiology of rabies in Britain is this: what is the probability that any particular control strategy would succeed in preventing the establishment of rabies if it were introduced into the fox population? The answer must depend a great deal on our knowledge of the demography and behaviour of foxes, and fortunately a good deal of very thorough work is being done in this country (cf. the chapters by D. W. Macdonald and H. G. Lloyd in Kaplan (1977)). These studies reveal a complex pattern of territorial behaviour, varying considerably with terrain and food supply. Typically, foxes live in family groups, each male having several vixens, of which only the dominant one will breed in a particular year. Births take place in the spring, and in the following autumn or later the young disperse, eventually to set up their own family groups. The existence of itinerant foxes means that territories vacated by resident foxes, or left vacant by their death, may be occupied quickly by itinerants, if not already absorbed into neighbouring territories. This is perhaps one of the reasons for the limited success of large-scale slaughtering policies in Europe.

Studies of fox behaviour reveal another interesting fact. Foxes are remarkably common in towns. This is true not only of lush suburban habitats, which often provide the best possible environment for the fox, but also of inner-city areas. This phenomenon could, of course, be very relevant to the possibility of a rabid dog infecting a fox before it dies.

Quantitative modelling

With this general background, I now want to discuss some of the considerations involved in the setting-up of a quantitative model of the disease. By a 'model' I mean a simplified description of the main features of the transmission, which by virtue of its simplification permits some rational and useful conclusions to be drawn about questions which otherwise might remain in dispute. By the word 'quantitative' I mean that the model is more than merely verbal; it involves numerical quantities which bear some resemblance to the real-life situation. The way in which conclusions are drawn may be mathematical, or it may be purely computational and hence involve the use of computers.

There is no unique model for rabies, any more than there is for any other disease. Different workers have proposed different approaches, often with rather different purposes in mind. As an aide-memoire I shall call these different approaches *descriptive, mechanistic* and *empirical*, although the use of any sort of label runs the risk of distorting the aims and achievements of particular authors.

Descriptive models

By a *descriptive* model I mean one for which the main purpose is to describe what is going on in as concise and evocative a manner as possible. As an example, let us consider some studies of the progress of the rabies front through Germany during the 1960s. If one examines maps showing locations of new cases of fox rabies year by year, the general drift westwards and southwards is clear. Yet it would be difficult from these maps alone to say exactly where the front was at any particular time. In a way, the problem is like one in communications engineering: there is a message but it is almost obscured by noise. It is perhaps no coincidence that some of the neatest work on data of this sort has been done by a communications engineer and his colleagues (Sayers *et al.*, 1977). Taking a particular region in southern Germany during the period 1963–71, they have effectively smoothed the irregular records of locations to provide a clearer visual message. By looking in detail at the changes from one time period to the next, they are able to trace the separate paths followed by the disease as it spread outwards from different foci. They show how the disease was held up for a time by the Danube and then proceeded along differentiated paths once the river had been crossed.

Another paper (Bögel *et al.*, 1976) provides a description of the same data from a rather different point of view.

Mechanistic models

The second category of models consists of those in which an attempt is made to build into the formal description elements simulating aspects of the transmission known to occur in reality. They are concerned with the *mechanism* of transmission. The elements might include the frequency of contacts between rabid and normal foxies, the distances moved by foxes, their demographic characteristics, the effect of control measures, and so on. The more complicated the model becomes, the less likely it is that progress can be made by purely mathematical means and the more likely it is that the investigator resorts to the computer. There is a temptation to move immediately towards detailed, complex models, and it is perhaps worth asking whether the mathematical theory of epidemics provides any general guidance not dependent on the mechanistic detail built into the model.

I mentioned earlier that a crucial question is whether, and under what circumstances, the disease would spread through the fox population if it were introduced. Suppose that one infected fox is introduced into a community of normal foxes. If it manages to transmit the disease to several other foxes before it dies, then the disease will have made a good start. If the initial fox dies before transmitting the disease, then that is the end of the matter. It turns out that the crucial question is how many new infections on the average are caused by direct transmission from one rabid fox. This quantity is called the *(net) reproduction rate*. If it is one or less the disease is bound to die out, although of course it may cause a small epidemic before doing so. If the reproduction rate exceeds one, there *is* a chance of the disease dying out, but there is now a real chance of it *growing* more or less indefinitely. Incidentally, only about half the rabid foxes have the 'furious' type of rabies, and the others are likely to be ineffective, so the furious foxes will need to have a reproduction rate greater than about two to ensure transmission. Now the reproduction rate depends on the biting habits of a rabid fox, on its period of infectivity before death, and on the density of susceptible foxes. Assuming the first two of these to be largely beyond our control, the possibility of reducing the reproduction rate seems to depend on that of reducing the density of susceptible foxes. Hence the policies of killing or immunizing a high proportion of the population. Unfortunately, it is quite difficult to estimate the reproduction rate that would obtain in any area, for little is known of the biting habits of rabid foxes. This is perhaps the biological feature which one would most like to measure in order to predict the chance that a threatened epidemic would take hold.

In many countries, elimination of rabies from animal populations is not an immediately feasible target, and the emphasis among field workers and modellers will be on reducing the intensity and the rate of spread. Suppose we are making observations at a point just ahead of the rabies front, and we count the number of new cases of fox rabies in a certain neighbourhood over successive periods of time. This number, the *incidence*, will rise as the epidemic is introduced into the neighbourhood. Then, after a while the incidence will fall because the stock of susceptibles becomes more and more depleted, until the disease disappears locally. The incidence thus takes the form of a wave passing through the neighbourhood leaving a trail of destruction behind it. This general phenomenon can be expressed mathematically. Moreover, it corresponds closely to what is seen in practice, for example in French and German data. The position of the front could be taken to be a boundary formed by some feature of this wave—for example, the maximum incidence. The question then arises—how quickly will it travel?

According to mathematical theory (Mollison, 1977) the speed of advance depends not only on the reproduction rate and incubation period, but also on the *contact distribution*: the distribution of the distance between the point at which any individual is infected and that at which this individual in turn causes a new infection. If these distances are usually large, the epidemic front will move relatively quickly. In practice we know little about the contact distances, which are caused in part by movements of rabid foxes. Following the tracks of a fox with rabies is not an exercise which commends itself to the average ethologist. Indeed, it may in practice be simplest to estimate these distances by reversing the argument—that is, by observing the speed of advance and thereby inferring properties of the contact distribution.

I am aware of six papers describing mechanistic models. One of these (Frerichs and Prawda, 1975) is concerned with transmission in urban dog populations in Colombia—a useful reminder that in many countries the disease is endemic in domestic animals, and that it is at least as much an urban as a rural problem. The authors remark that "in Colombia, a democracy with a history of internal violence, a canine euthanasia campaign would be politically unacceptable".

They make various assumptions about the movements of rabid dogs, their contact with normal dogs, the migration into and out of the system, and the effect of vaccination. They then assess the effect of different vaccination policies, taking cost into account. They recommend a policy in which vaccination teams move about the city, concentrating their efforts in parts of the city where the density of susceptible dogs is highest.

The other models (Berger, 1976; Grant, 1977, Lambinet *et al.*, 1978; Preston, 1973; Smart and Giles, 1973) deal with fox rabies. They make different assumptions about such features as latent and infectious periods, contact rates, movement of foxes, and the birth and death rates. All except Lambinet *et al.* incorporate random variation in various ways, and results are obtained by computer simulations. Such models, incorporating random elements, are called *stochastic*. They have the merit of allowing these chance elements to play their part in determining the course of events—as they do in practice—but the corollary is that one run through the system (or *realization*) is not enough evidence on which to assess the range of possible outcomes. The process must be repeated several times, and a computer is normally essential.

Some of the results obtained by these authors show qualitative features which could perhaps have been predicted by simpler means. In some of the models a range of values for certain parameters, such as fox density, is explored, and it is noted that for some values, e.g., high densities, the disease is maintained, whereas for others, low densities, it tends to die out. This is largely a matter of the reproduction rate discussed earlier, and some detailed work needs to be done to check that the observed threshold phenomenon accords with what we should expect in theory.

Some authors have incorporated seasonal effects into their models (for example in fox reproduction, dispersal and death). These naturally produce annual fluctuations in rabies incidence (which in practice is highest in the early part of the year). If the simulated epidemic were continued sufficiently long, there might be the opportunity to see whether longer cycles were suggested. In real data, cycles of 3 to 5 years have been reported. The reason presumably is that a reduction in fox population is caused by the disease and it takes several years for the numbers to build up again. The simulations are suggestive but not conclusive on this point, mainly, I think, because the simulated time period has been too short.

Lambinet *et al.* (1978) adopt a somewhat different approach, with a largely deterministic model leading to a set of mathematical equations which are solved by means of a computer. Their concern is mainly short-term. They are able to reproduce the shape of the epidemic wave mentioned earlier, and they claim to have chosen parameter values which provide a realistic value for the speed of advance.

The main problem facing the mechanistic modeller is to know what to assume about the movement and biting habits of foxes. It seems likely that these are affected by terrain, habitat and fox density, and little is known about the nature of these effects. Is it, for example, possible that a control policy of killing foxes in an area in which rabies is being transmitted enables any surviving rabid foxes to travel greater distances and hence to *increase* the rate of advance? It is mathematically possible, and perhaps one of the tasks facing the modeller is to explain to the control authorities the circumstances under which this paradoxical consequence might or might not occur.

A further problem is that most mathematical models for disease processes assume homogeneous conditions over the whole population, whereas in practice the picture is very much more patchy. For example, there will be some subgroups of the population with much higher contact rates than the average because the individuals are closer together. In some respects these fluctuations average out, but in other ways they are likely to be quite important. For example, it would be possible for a fox population to show an average reproduction rate of less than one, and yet for transmission to continue because in some subgroups the rate exceeds one. Future modelling exercises will probably have to allow for heterogeneity of this sort.

Empirical models

A third approach to the quantitative study of rabies epidemiology, which I have called *empirical*, is to rely more on the statistical analysis of data and less on the deductions to be drawn from an axiomatic model. Suppose it were possible to make observations at a number of points along the present rabies front, stretching for several hundred miles and covering a wide range of environmental conditions. At each point one would try to measure the intensity of transmission locally—whether or not it dies out, and, if not, the speed of advance. One would also measure a number of possible explanatory factors—variables which might affect transmission, such as fox density, nature of terrain, habitat and food supply, local control measures, etc. One would then do a statistical analysis to see to what extent the transmission variables could be predicted by the explanatory variables. If there was little evidence of correlation, there would be a need to review the set of assumptions underlying both modelling exercises and actual control policy. If there were a correlation, there would be at least some prospect of predicting the likelihood of transmission in other areas. This programme is idealistic in that the necessary measurements probably cannot easily be made. Fox densities, for example, are not generally available. It seems to me, though, worth considering the feasibility of this sort of study, and perhaps doing some work on a pilot scale. As it happens, there is a programme of collaborative European research on rabies, co-ordinated by Dr. K. Bögel of the World Health Organization, which may well be able to work along these lines.

Conclusion

The study of quantitative models for the transmission of rabies has not yet provided control authorities with any clear-cut advice about the relative effectiveness of different control measures. It has, however, stimulated some careful thought about possible 'scenarios', and has highlighted some of the quantities which play an essential role in transmission and yet are hard to measure. Mathematicians and statisticians by themselves are unlikely to make significant progress, but the growing collaboration between these groups and the biological specialists is most welcome and in my view holds promise for the future.

Acknowledgements

Much of the content of this paper has been influenced by discussions with members of the Working Party on Quantitative Studies in the Epidemiology of Rabies which is supported by the

Royal Statistical Society and the Institute of Terrestrial Ecology. I have benefited especially from recent discussions with Mr. F. Ball, Dr. J. F. Boisvieux, Dr. D. W. Macdonald and Dr. D. Mollison.

References

BAILEY, N. T. J. (1975) *The Mathematical Theory of Infectious Diseases.* London: Griffin.

BERGER, J. (1976) Model of rabies control. In *Mathematical Models in Medicine, Lecture Notes in Biomathematics, No. 11,* eds. BERGER, J., BÜHLER, W., REPGES, R. and TAUTU, P. Berlin: Springer-Verlag.

BÖGEL, K., MOEGLE, H., KNORPP, F., ARATA, A., DIETZ, K. and DIETHELM, P. (1976) Characteristics of the spread of wildlife rabies epidemic in Europe. *Bulletin of the World Health Organization,* **54,** 433-447.

COHEN, J. E. (1977) Mathematical models of schistosomiasis. *Annual Review of Ecology and Systematics,* **8,** 209-233.

FRERICHS, R. R. and PRAWDA, J. (1975) A computer simulation model for the control of rabies in an urban area of Colombia. *Management Science.* **22,** 411-421.

GRANT. G. C. (1977) A simulation study of a red fox population with rabies. M.A. Thesis, Queens University, Kingston, Ontario, Canada.

KAPLAN, C. (ed.) (1977) *Rabies: the Facts.* London: Oxford University Press.

LAMBINET, D., BOISVIEUX, J.-F., MALLET, A., ARTOIS, M. and ANDRAL, L. (1978) Modèle mathématique de la propagation d'une épizootie de rage vulpine. *Revue d'Epidémiologie et de Santé Publique,* **26,** 9-28.

LLOYD, H. G. (1977) Wildlife rabies: prospects of Britain. In Kaplan (1977), pp. 91-103.

MACDONALD, D. W. (1977) The behavioural ecology of the red fox. In Kaplan (1977), pp. 70-90.

MACDONALD, G. (1973) *Dynamics of Tropical Disease.* London: Oxford University Press.

MOLLISON. D. (1977) Spatial contact models for ecological and epidemic spread. *Journal of the Royal Statistical Society,* B, **39,** 283-326.

PRESTON. E. M. (1973) Computer simulated dynamics of a rabies-controlled fox population. *Journal of Wildlife Management.* **37,** 501-512.

SAYERS, B. McA., MANSOURIAN, B. G., PHAN TAN, T. and BÖGEL, K. (1977) A pattern-analysis study of a wild-life rabies epizootic. *Medical Informatics,* **2,** 11-34.

SCHWABE, C. W. (1971) *Report of 1st WHO seminar on veterinary public health, Mukteswar, India.* New Delhi: World Health Organization.

SMART, C. W. and GILES, R. H. JR. (1973) A computer model of wildlife rabies epizootics and an analysis of incidence patterns. *Wildlife Diseases,* **61,** 1-89.

URBANIZATION AND STRESS

G. AINSWORTH HARRISON

Department of Biological Anthropology, University of Oxford

STRESS is a word used with various meanings. Many of the components of the stress concept are embraced by saying that stress is a change in homeostatic systems which, if persistent, threatens an individual's fitness. Unfortunately, such a definition introduces a further term of some complexity: 'fitness'; but for many purposes this can be equated with health — if that helps! There is also an element of tautology in the definition, since homeostasis itself and health can amount to the same thing. However, there are many settings of homeostatic mechanisms which are compatible with good health or high fitness. The important positive components of the definition are that it refers to a state of the person, not to a state of the environment (for an environmental factor which produces stress in one individual may not in another); and that it is always a harmful or potentially harmful condition, never beneficial. One can thus, on this definition, never have 'too little' stress. If physical exercise is typically beneficial then the physiological responses to it are not stresses. On the other hand, the definition does permit consideration of diseases which are not normally regarded as stress diseases — as for example the effects of infectious diseases, though of course these can be excluded by *caveat*.

Measuring Stress in Terms of Fitness

With this view of stress, there appear to be four main ways in which it can be measured.

(1) In terms of its effects on mortality/longevity and, in some instances fertility. These are clearly related to overall reproductive success or Darwinian fitness — the parameter of evolutionary concern, and the most general concept of fitness. The data required for analyses are typically available on whole populations from censuses and the like, and can be used for examining the effects on different subgroups of a population living under different environmental conditions.

(2) In terms of its effects on morbidity, including mental morbidity. Since there is an obvious connection between morbidity and mortality, this approach is also connected, though loosely, with reproductive success as well as health. The data are typically collected through health services and medical surveys and can often be analysed on a more individual basis than can that obtained through routine demographic censuses.

(3) In terms of its effects on well-being and day-to-day functioning of individuals. Although examination of such effects is clearly related to studies of morbidity, I distinguish it from such studies because the concern is with people's subjective evaluation of themselves, and this may not involve any objectively diagnosable pathology. It also requires intensive interviews and detailed questionnaires to establish, and there are many other methodological problems.

(4) In terms of the effects of stress on the physiology and endocrinology of people actually experiencing the stress at the time of investigation. This is far removed from reproductive success, but it attempts to measure the other side of the definitional coin — the change in homeostatic systems. Much of the work is done experimentally in laboratories with scientific controls, but the approach can and has been applied in field situations.

When we come to consider the particular issue of the stresses arising from the urbanization of man, it is of course necessary not only to measure stress levels but also to relate them to those found in other environmental situations. This raises the question of whether a set of base levels can be meaningfully recognized. Account has also to be taken of the fact that urbanization itself is a highly heterogeneous phenomenon, and not only are there marked differences between urbanization in the developed and developing worlds, but also from one city to another, and indeed from one small part of some city to another. Further, it is likely that different cultural practices, traditions and expectations will strongly influence the extent to which any particular environmental agent produces a stress. Other problems of comparability arise from coincidental factors, especially in temporal analyses. Cases of attempted suicide, for example, appear to have risen dramatically in Britain since the war (Mills and Eden, 1976), but at least some of this change is likely to be due to the greater ease with which suicide can be attempted when various lethal drugs are readily available.

On the question of base levels, it has been suggested, particularly by Boyden (1970) that since hominids practised a hunter–gatherer type of existence for most of their evolution, it is to a Palaeolithic life-style that man is genetically adapted. Boyden (1972) has itemized the dramatic changes which have occurred since this life-style has been abandoned by most populations, in physical, chemical, nutritional, epidemiological and social environments, and predicts that evidence of what he terms 'phylogenetic maladjustment' should be detectable in modern societies. On the basis of this argument, one might expect that the levels of stress experienced by modern 'hunter–gatherers' would constitute 'base levels'. However, present hunter–gatherers with a truly traditional life-style are rare; they are in many ways unrepresentative of general Palaeolithic populations, particularly in being confined to especially hazardous environments; and little is known of their stress levels, however it is measured. Because of the marked qualitative as well as quantitative differences between hunter–gatherers and modern urban populations, it is also doubtful whether any overall measure of stress would be meaningful. Nevertheless, I propose to consider the evidence such as it is and also examine data from other types of traditional societies, such as subsistence cultivators, who retain features of earlier life-styles.

More useful from the comparative viewpoint are the differences between urban groups and surrounding rural populations, especially when, as is usual, these have the same cultural traditions and expectations. In most situations, and invariably in the developed world, rural communities have been profoundly influenced by neighbouring towns and cities and by general features of urbaniz-ation. In this, however, the environmental factors involved are typically of lesser degree, as for example in pollution, noise, crowding and anomie, and this allows the examination of some of their effects. Similar comparisons are possible and useful within cities themselves, for as already mentioned there is marked heterogeneity in many environmental factors from one part of any city to another. In addition, within cities environmental factors of importance can vary somewhat independently of one another, which allows some partitioning of effects.

I shall now attempt to examine the four types of stress measurement in the three types of contrasting situation: (a) modern hunter–gatherer and traditional societies versus urban societies; (b) urban versus rural; and (c) within-city heterogeneity.

Mortality/Longevity Measures

So far as the first contrast is concerned, most of the useful data relate to the demographic measures. Howell (1976) estimates that for the !Kung-speaking San, expectation of life at birth is about 30 years with about 23 per cent of infants dying in the first year of life, 40 per cent of people dying before they reach 15, 60 per cent before the age of 45 and with only 15 per cent of new-borns surviving to live to 65. Similar figures have been obtained for other hunter–gatherer groups (Birdsell, 1972), and among the Yanomama, largely because of female infanticide, the life expectancy at birth is as low as 20 years (Neel and Weiss, 1975). For prehistoric populations, Acsádi and Nemeskéri (1970) have estimated that life expectancy at birth for *Homo erectus* was less than 20 years and in the Magkreb-type of the Neolithic in the low twenties. These levels of life expectancy are, of course, extremely low by comparison with modern industrialized countries. In England and Wales in 1971, for example, male life expectancy at birth was 69 years and female life expectancy 75. The levels were a little lower in Scotland. Even in 1871 the comparable figures were around 42 and 45 (Howe, 1972). However, the general abandonment of hunter–gathering and the beginnings of urbanization are, of course, much earlier than this, and life expectation throughout classical and mediaeval times appears to have been comparable with prehistoric levels. Thus figures of 22 for Roman Egypt, 35 for 13th century Englishmen, 33·5 for late 17th century inhabitants of Breslau and 35·5 for mid-18th century New Englanders are cited by Weiner (1977). It is widely stated that urban populations in the early stages of the industrial revolution in England were unable to maintain themselves and required constant replenishment from surrounding rural populations. The main factor in the dramatic increase in longevity in modern times in the developed world is, of course, the increasing control and elimination of infectious disease, although the way this was initially effected is still a matter of some controversy (McKeown and Lowe, 1977). In the developing world, life expectancy is still low; in India for example, 41·9 for males and 40·5 for females in 1951–60 (*Demographic Yearbook*, 1976).

The current urban–rural contrasts are more meaningful. The data for England and Wales in 1971 show a very clear relationship between stillbirths and infant deaths and the size of the place of residence of the parents, ranging from 31·7/thousand births for conurbations to 27·0/thousand for rural districts. This advantage of rural residence, particularly in males, is evidenced in all subsequent age groups. Thus the ratio of death rates for males in conurbations versus rural districts is 0·53/0·51 in the 1–14 year olds, 1·39/1·37 in 15–44 year olds, 14·40/11·76 in the 45–64 year olds and 79·76/70·76 in those who are 65 and above (H.M.S.O., 1973). Similar trends occur in other developed countries, as for example Denmark and the Netherlands, but the phenomenon is not universal. In the developing world, e.g., Pakistan, death rates may be greater in rural areas at practically all ages, but especially in the very young (*Demographic Yearbook*, 1976). This, no doubt, is mainly due to the concentration of scarce medical resources in urban centres.

As a good example of the demographic analysis of differential stress within cities, one can site the recent study of Herzog, Levy and Verdonk (1976) on Rotterdam. These authors examined, by multiple regression analysis, patterns of what they term 'pathology' within different sections of the city in relation to possible determinants, such as measures of crowding, social stability, social homogeneity, social class, quality of housing and population structure. Among various 'dependent' characteristics they include age-adjusted total mortality rate, perinatal deaths and infant deaths. They found that total death rate showed some relationship with crowding and with the amount of migration (taken as a measure of social stability). Patterns of infant and perinatal death, however, showed little if any relationship with the independent variables, which in a city like Rotterdam with well developed social and medical facilities is probably not surprising.

Morbidity measures

Turning now to morbidity as the measure of stress, it is practically impossible to compare present-day hunter–gatherer patterns with those for modern urban groups, since the epidemiological situations are so qualitatively different and do not allow a meaningful comparison. It has been pointed out by Boyden and others that the great increase in population size, which started with the Neolithic but which has been largely associated with urbanization, greatly changed host–parasite relations. Thus it has been shown how measles must be a relatively new disease of man because of its need of access to large numbers of people (Fenner, 1970) and Boyden suggests that the increase in world population may be leading to an evolutionary adaptive radiation of many viruses. However, hunter–gatherers typically have high levels of infection with parasitic worms and protozoan pathogens. What does seem certain and important is that hunter–gatherers and other peoples with traditional life style have very low levels of cardiovascular disease, and do not show the increase in blood pressure with age which is so much a feature of modern industrialized societies. Blood pressure changes may be extremely sensitive to stress, for Day, Bailey and Robinson (1979) have shown that Maasai who have only recently abandoned their traditional way of life and are still living close to it show a chronic increase in blood pressure.

Various studies have indicated remarkably high levels of severe disablement through mental illness in modern Western societies (Lader, 1975). About a quarter of the adult populations of London and New York (Srole *et al.*, 1962) experience some illness which is diagnosed as entirely psychiatric in nature, and less than 20 per cent are devoid of symptoms of emotional disturbance. Cross-cultural comparisons even for moderately discrete and severe conditions are not easy and there are no reliable data for hunter–gatherer societies. However, Leighton *et al.* (1963 a) found comparable levels of mental ill health in a traditional society in rural Nigeria to those reported for London and New York, and this was probably not due to differences in diagnosis, as the same group found high levels also in rural Canada (Leighton *et al.*, 1963 b). Social anthropologists have also commented on the substantial incidence of mental illness in traditional societies. What certainly differs between the traditional and developed world is how the mentally sick are treated medically and by society.

The comparison of urban and rural groups for morbidity is again more helpful. Rose (1976) has made a compilation of the rates of a number of diseases in England and Wales in 1971 by the size of the place of residence. For various conditions related to droplet-borne infections — respiratory tuberculosis, rheumatic heart disease, measles during the first year of life, and G.P. consultations for the common cold, the incidence is notably higher in conurbations than in rural districts. Towns of intermediate size tend to have intermediate levels. Much of this difference arises from varying levels of crowding, but coronary heart disease also shows a similar pattern of incidence (see Affluence, urbanization and coronary heart disease, by M. G. Marmot; pp. 127–143).

When we come to consider mental illness, there are some special problems of interpretation, the main ones being variable diagnosis and mental health affecting one's place of residence. Nevertheless, the fact that consultations for psychoneurotic disorders in Britain average 32/1000 for conurbations and only 23 for rural districts (Logan and Cushion, 1958), with towns of intermediate size tending to be intermediate in status, probably reflects a real urban–rural difference. Consultations for peptic ulcer, which has a high psychosomatic component in its aetiology, show a similar distributional pattern, as do all consultations related to 'emotional stress'. The figures for these are extremely high, 610/1000/year for conurbations and 567/1000/year for rural districts (Logan and Cushion, 1958). On the other hand, little or no difference in psychoneurotic morbidity prevalence was observed between the populations of an old dilapidated city centre, a piece of suburbia and a recent new town development (Taylor and Chave, 1964), but again rates were high. In this study, neurotic symptoms were about twice as common in females as in males and formally diagnosed anxiety states constituted about half of all the psychoneurotic symptoms. Susceptibility did not relate to income or length of residence in the particular type of environment. Salkind (1973) also found that 44 per cent of the UK population were "anxious", with anxiety scores increasing with age and in lower social groups. He did not, however, detect urban–rural differences, although high prevalences were found in East Anglia, West Midlands and South Wales.

Over-all, the evidence does indicate a higher physical and mental morbidity in cities and towns than in surrounding rural areas, but the differences in most cases are not great and are often exceeded by regional variations (Howe, 1976). For some "conditions", the difference is the other way round, e.g. major traffic accidents. Even after standardization for age effects, many pathologies show marked patterns of variation within cities. Some of these patterns are quite clearly related to patterns in the physical environment such as air pollution, but others have no clear causation. In the Rotterdam study already cited (Herzog et al., 1976), mental hospital admissions were related to geographical variation in density, population heterogeneity and social class, but suicide patterns did not follow significantly the distribution of any of the independent variables examined. In an intensive study of the geographical distribution within Chicago of admissions into mental institutions, Levy and Rowitz (1973) found considerable variations by housing district, and particularly by the rateable value of property. The males admittedly tended to come from the lowest socio-economic areas, but this may have been due to the downward social mobility of people as they become mentally ill. Incidentally, Levy and Rowitz found higher rates of male than female admission, under-representation in the patients of those who were under 25 years of age, proportionally more black patients from areas where there were few black residents, and a high level of susceptibility in those who were single, widowed, separated or divorced.

Most of the studies of the morbidity effects of urban life have not been so geographically based. Rather the approach has been to take some single environmental factor or group of factors, which if not unique to cities is quantitatively different in them, and examine its effects either experimentally or by comparing groups that contrast maximally. The experimental approach has been very useful for analysing such discrete variables as noise — revealing that high noise levels generally reduce the performance of various physical and psychological tests, except when the subject is fatigued, when performance may be raised by moderate noise (Broadbent, 1976) — but this approach is largely limited to the examination of acute effects, and is much more difficult to manipulate with complex features of the social environment.

When studies are conducted on a population basis there are many methodological problems. One of the most serious of these is the high level of intercorrelation between many environmental factors. High levels of crowding, for example, are frequently associated with economic poverty and low levels of education. Because of this, there is disagreement about the consequences of crowding as such, but the general conclusion of Freedman (1975) on reviewing the extensive literature is that "people who live under crowded conditions do not suffer from being crowded". Certainly in some societies high levels of crowding are the norm, e.g., in Hong Kong. However, in Hong Kong, Millar (1976) claims to have shown that high physical density is associated with what she terms biopsychic maladjustment.

The phenomenon of crowding also exemplifies the problem of identifying the most useful units of measurement. Jalle, Cove and McPherson (1972) used four different measures of density: number of persons per room; number of persons per housing unit; number of housing units per housing structure; and number of structures per hectare. Psychiatric disorders correlated most highly with numbers of persons per housing unit, while the incidence of children in care and 'aggressive acts' were associated with room density. The other two measures showed little relationship with the 'morbidity' examined, yet they are the ones which specifically categorize urban conditions.

A behavioural feature which tends to characterize all advanced societies but is particularly evidenced in those who live and work in cities is a high level of individual mobility. This is found both in daily activity and in the frequency of house moves, and of course involves what from the evolutionary point of view is quite novel, the use of mechanical transport — mobility without physical effort. Apart from the travel itself, there are also important ramifying consequences such as the coming into fleeting contact with large numbers of other people who are not known in any permanent social context, and the geographical dispersion of kin-groups. As far as I am aware, however, there is no information on the effects of mobility and the means of mobility on morbidity patterns, except, of course, on traffic accidents. One might reasonably infer from numerous investigations on the effects of physical exercise that those who walk to work and in work will be in many respects, especially cardiovascular features, healthier than those who use cars and trains.

While, surprisingly, so little is known about travel effects, it has been shown (Holmes and Rahe, 1967; Ruben, Gunderson and Arthur, 1971) that the frequency of 'life events' is positively correlated with susceptibility to both physical and mental illness. Interestingly, this is so whether the life events are undesired or desired ones. Life events are probably most common in urban societies, but there are difficulties in interpretation, since what may constitute an important life event to one person may be inconsequential to another.

Measures of well-being

The problems of interpretation become persistently acute when we try to examine subjective assessments of well-being as the measure of stress. Indeed, even the value scale can be a matter of debate. Few would dispute that having a duodenal ulcer was a morbid state, but how about the taking of pleasurable drugs? There can also frequently be a conflict between an individual's values and society's values. A successful criminal may well be very satisfied with life, but society regards a high crime rate as undesirable. It is not in my province to examine the nature of stress in a social system as a whole, but 'social deviance' has been considered as an element of individual stress.

Another problem concerns interpretation of what people say, especially in response to questionnaires. It is very evident from many studies that a substantial proportion of people when asked about their own emotions and feelings give answers which they judge are the ones which the interviewer wishes to hear or the ones which are most socially acceptable. Even if they express their 'real' feelings, what are these? Clearly they vary from time to time in most people and at best only have a probabilistic 'truth'.

Because of difficulties of this kind I doubt if it is possible to compare subjective satisfaction levels of peoples in different cultures. Many anthropologists have commented on the 'happiness' of hunter-gatherers like the Bushman and Pygmy, but it is doubtful if this has much scientific validity and one notices that few of these anthropologists have attempted to transfer permanently to these societies!

The position is potentially more tractable in urban–rural contrasts, but there are few reliable data as yet. Because of the intrinsic methodological difficulties, it is not meaningful to cross-compare the results of different investigations. A case where one researcher has examined both rural and urban groups by the same techniques is that of Millar (1976) in Hong Kong. She finds that the rural group report a higher frequency of well-being. In our own survey of Oxfordshire villages, many of the inhabitants work in towns and cities. In a pilot analysis of levels of satisfaction, boredom, frustration, etc., we have found little relationship with occupation, except that farmers and other agricultural groups seem more contented with the quality of their lives than do other groups. They can probably be regarded as having the least urbanized life-style. More reliable than what people say, is what they do. People in cities are less likely to help strangers in trouble (Oates, 1974). This may be due in part to the fact that people are less likely to communicate with strangers when there are other people present (Darley and Latane, 1968), and it does appear that loneliness is a particularly severe problem in cities (Reiseman, 1950).

So far as social deviance is concerned, Rutter (1973) found that 'conduct disorder' as well as neurotic symptoms were strikingly more frequent among young schoolchildren in an inner London suburb than on the Isle of Wight. The disturbed children in both places tended to come from unhappy homes, but these were commoner in London.

Various urban studies have shown important associations between social deviance and such factors as poverty, poor housing and few amenities, large family size, poor parental behaviours and low intelligence (Shaw and MacKay, 1942; Wallis and Maliphant, 1967; West, 1973), but causal connections are difficult to disentangle. All these, however, are factors which are likely to occur in modern urban situations. In a specific examination of housing, Wing (1974) concludes that high-rise apartments had a deleterious effect on children, especially pre-school children, but considerable levels of dissatisfaction were expressed by people in all sorts of housing. Drug dependence, and smoking and drinking by children, are particularly likely to develop where subcultures arise which reinforce deviant behaviour by attaching high value to it (Wing, 1976). In the developed world the structure of cities seems to provide just the sort of conditions for such subcultures to develop. How far we can regard the patterns of socially deviant behaviours as signs of stress is a matter of debate, as I have already said, but that there are many serious problems arising out of the form of urban societies can hardly be denied.

Endocrinological measures

When we come to consider the levels of stress hormones as a measure of stress, we are no longer directly concerned with changes in fitness. Indeed we can view the output of stress hormones as a means of attempting to maintain a constant fitness under environmental change. Of course, if homeostasis cannot be maintained by the physiological and endocrinological systems, than a fall in fitness will ensue. Further, mere excessive invoking of an 'adaptive response' may lead to pathology, particularly if this occurs in situations for which it was not genetically programmed by evolution. The catecholamine 'flight–fight' response must have been advantageous to Palaeolithic hunters, but there is evidence that if it is repeatedly evoked in circumstances where it is not associated with high levels of physical exercise it can be an important component in the aetiology of coronary heart disease (Carruthers, 1976).

While there is evidence that growth hormone (Greenwood and Landon, 1966), prolactin (Frantz, Kleinberg and Noel, 1972), and thyroid hormones (Mason, 1972) can be regarded as stress hormones, I will confine this short review to consideration of the adrenocorticoid hormones, particularly the glucocorticoids, and the catecholamines. Their role in stress has been extensively reviewed by Mason (1972).

There is strong evidence that 17-ketosteroid output levels are higher in peoples in technologically advanced societies, than in those living more traditional life-styles in Nigeria (Barnicot and Wolffson, 1952), South Africa (Politzer and Tucker, 1958), India (Friedman, 1954) and China (Ch'en Peien, 1956). Allbrook (1956) has also found that the size of the adrenal cortex in East African males is less than in white Americans. It has been noted that all these non-Western peoples live in the tropics and it has been surmised that their low ketosteroid levels may be due to nutritional and climatic factors. Barnicot and Wolffson (1952) showed, however, that there were no detectable differences in steroid metabolism between Nigerians and Londoners, and it could well be that life-style is an important determinant of the differences. Barnicot and Wolffson found that Nigerians in London tended to preserve the African pattern. There do not appear to be any comparable data for catecholamines—a situation which is in need of remedy.

Data for urban–rural comparisons are also not available, but it is of some relevance that in our field study of Oxfordshire villages (Jenner, Reynolds and Harrison, 1979) we found quite marked differences in adrenaline output on workdays between those with manual occupations and those with non-manual ones. The latter had the higher levels.

Although whole-population data on stress hormones are still very sparse, knowledge of the effects of particular environmental situations, behaviours and emotional states is now increasing rapidly. Experiences such as competitive sport (Hill *et al.*, 1956), expeditions (Simpson, 1967), hospitalization (Hamburg, 1962), battle (Howard *et al.*, 1955), interviews (Persky *et al.*, 1958), examinations (Hamburg, 1962), and sleep deprivation (Mason, 1959) have been monitored for their effects on 17-hydroxycorticosteroid secretion and/or excretion. There are also considerable data on experimental animals examining the effects of housing and social organization (Mason, 1959). Similarly the effects on catecholamine output of hospital admission (Tolson *et al.*, 1965), sleep deprivation (Metz, Schaff and Grivel, 1960), examinations (Bogdonoff *et al.*, 1960), violent films (Euler *et al.*, 1959), piecework (Levi, 1964), commuting (Lundberg, 1976) etc. have seen studied. Typically the conditions cited raise the levels of stress hormone output.

Many of these conditions are part of daily life in the modern world and though not strictly urban they are very much a part of the experience of the city dweller. It is hard to generalize over all the results which have been reported, but it does seem that the psychological factors are at least as important, and are probably much more important than the physical factors in determining these responses. To take just one example, the cox in a boat race showed just as great an increase in 17-hydroxycorticosteroids as did the rowers.

Kety (1962) notes that the experimental administration of adrenaline is associated with mental states variously described as anxiety, apprehensiveness, excitement, tenseness, exhilaration, restlessness, agitation or fear. Experimental subjects note however, that it is "as if they were experiencing these emotions". There seems little doubt that the originating site of them normally is in the CNS and that from there they cause the secretion of adrenaline. They are all likely to be experienced when individuals or groups find it difficult or impossible "to anticipate future events in their social environments". This, according to Groen and Bastiaans (1975), is a central feature of Western society, which they further say is characterized by "complicated, randomized and contradictory psychosocial signals" as compared with traditional societies. These features are likely to be accentuated in urban groups and it would be surprising if it is not shown that adrenaline and probably noradrenaline output is not also increased in urban environments, particularly when people are living outside structured communities.

Conclusions

This review has covered only a very small part of the extensive literature relevant to analysing urbanization and stress (but I hope the coverage has been representative and balanced). Even so, there are innumerable major deficiencies in our knowledge, particularly for the developing world. The evidence, such as it is, does suggest particularly from the urban–rural comparisons that city residents in the developed world are at greater 'risk' from stress, but on the objective scales, at least, this is not a dramatic phenomenon. Further, many of the situations which generate stress are as much a part of the nature of Western development as of urbanization as such, and at least some of the differences between urban and rural groups are likely to be due to the varying levels to which they have been affected by development. Many of the really damaging factors, like poverty, are clearly not inevitable correlates of urbanization or development.

Despite some recent attempts to glorify life-styles in traditional societies, there is little objective evidence to warrant this. They generate their own problems for both physical and mental health and trading off cardiovascular disease for uncertain nutrition is a questionable gain. For most people 'quantity of life' in terms of longevity is not an unimportant component of the 'quality of life'.

Whatever the merits of traditional and rural societies, the one thing we can be reasonably certain of is that an ever increasing proportion of the world's population is going to be living in cities. At the moment about 17 per cent of people live in 'metros' and on present trends the proportion will rise to 50 per cent by the year 2000 (Dentler, 1977). Such problems of stress as are indeed associated with urbanization must, therefore, clearly be resolved within the framework of cities themselves: a return to the land is just 'not on' for more than a few, whatever its advantages. It is therefore going to be increasingly important to try to find ways of incorporating within the structure of cities, social as well as physical features which mitigate stress. Perhaps it will turn out that the most useful thing that can be learned from traditional societies and the evolutionary perspective is the value of the 'small scale' in human relations. Living and working in situations where there are strong kith and kin support systems may well be the most important way to protect from stress or alleviate it when it does occur. It should not be beyond the wit of the planners to build up the large scale through the small scale.

References

ACSÁDI, G. and NEMESKÉRI, J. (1970) *History of Human Life Span and Mortality.* Budapest: Akadémiai Kiado.

ALLBROOK, D. (1956) Size of adrenal cortex in East African males. *Lancet*, 606–687.

BARNICOT, N. A. and WOLFFSON, D. (1952) Daily urinary 17-ketosteroid output of African Negroes. *Lancet*, 893–894.

BIRDSELL, J. B. (1972) *Human Evolution: An Introduction to the New Physical Anthropology.* Chicago: Rand McNally.

BOGDONOFF, M. D., ESTES, E. H., HARLAN, W. R., TROUT, D. L. and KIRSHNER, N. (1960) Metabolic and cardiovascular changes during a state of acute central nervous system arousal. *Journal of Clinical Endocrinology*, **20**, 1333–1340.

BOYDEN, S. V. (1972) Ecology in relation to urban population structure. In *The Structure of Human Populations*, eds. HARRISON, G. A. and BOYCE, A. J. Oxford: Oxford University Press.

BOYDEN, S. V. (Ed.) (1970) *The Impact of Civilization on the Biology of Man.* Toronto: University of Toronto Press.

BROADBENT, D. E. (1976) Environment and performance in man. In *Urban Environments*, eds. HARRISON, G. A. and GIBSON, J. B. Oxford: Oxford University Press.

CARRUTHERS, M. (1976) Biochemical responses to environmental stress in man. In *Urban Environments*, Eds. HARRISON, G. A. and GIBSON, J. B. Oxford: Oxford University Press.

CH'EN PEIEN (1956) *Chinese Medical Journal*, **74**, 424, cited in POLITZER, W. M. and TUCKER, B. (1958) *loc. cit.*

DARLEY, J. M. and LATANE, B. (1968) Bystander intervention in emergencies: diffusion of responsibility. *Journal of Personality and Social Psychology*, **8**, 377–383.

DAY, J., BAILEY, A. and ROBINSON, D. (1979) Biological variations associated with changes in lifestyle among the pastoral and nomadic tribes of East Africa. *Annals of Human Biology*, **6**, 29–39.

Demographic Yearbook (1976) 28th Issue. New York: United Nations.

DENTLER, R. A. (1977) *Urban Problems.* Chicago: Rand McNally.

EULER, U. S., GEMZELL, C. A., LEVI, L. and STROM, G. (1959) Cortical and medullary adrenal activity in emotional stress. *Acta Endocrinologica*, **30**, 567–573.

FENNER, F. (1970) The effects of changing social organization on the infectious diseases of man. In *The Impact of Civilization on the Biology of Man*, ed. BOYDEN, S. V. Toronto: University of Toronto Press.

FRANTZ, A. G., KLEINBERG, D. and NOEL, G. L. (1972) Prolactin studies in man. *Recent Progress in Hormone Research*, **28**, 527–590.

FREEDMAN, J. L. (1975) *Crowding and Behaviour: The Psychology of High Density Living.* New York: The Viking Press.

FRIEDMAN, H. C. (1954) Urinary ketosteroids in Indian males. *Lancet*, 262–266.

GREENWOOD, F. C. and LANDON, J. (1966) Growth hormone secretion in response to stress in man. *Nature*, **210**, 540–541.

GROEN, J. J. and BASTIAANS, J. (1975) Psychosocial stress, interhuman communication and psychosomatic disease. In *Stress and Anxiety*, ed. SPIELBERGER, C. D. and SARASON, I. G. New York: John Wiley & Sons.

HAMBURG, D. A. (1962) Plasma and urinary corticosteroid levels in naturally occurring psychological stresses. *Research Publications of the Association for Research in Nervous and Mental Diseases*, **40**, 406–413.

HERZOG, A. N., LEVY, L. and VERDONK, A. (1976) Some ecological factors associated with health and social adaptation in the city of Rotterdam. *Urban Ecology*, **2**, 205–234.

HILL, S. R., GOETZ, F. C., FOX, H. M., MURANSKI, B. J., KRAKAVER, L. J., REIFENSTEIN, R. W., GRAY, S. J., REDDY, W. J., HEDBERG, S. E., ST. MARC, J. R. and THORN, G. W. (1956) Studies on adrenocortical and psychological response to stress in man. *Archives of Internal Medicine*, **97**, 269–298.

H.M.S.O. (1973) *Registrar General's Statistical Review of England and Wales for 1971* London: H.M.S.O.

HOLMES, T. H. and RAHE, R. H. (1967) The social re-adjustment rating scale. *Journal of Psychosomatic Research*, **11**, 213–218.

HOWARD, J. M., OLNEY, J. M., FRAWLEY, J. P., PETERSON, R. E., SMITH, L. H., DAVIS, J. H., GUERRA, S. and DIBRELL, W. H. (1955) Studies of adrenal function in combat and wounded soldiers. *Annals of Surgery*, **141**, 314–320.

HOWE, G. M. (1972) *Man, Environment and Disease in Britain*. Newton Abbot: David & Charles.

HOWE, G. M. (1976) Aspects of medical geography in Great Britain. In *Man in Urban Environments*, ed. HARRISON, G. A. and GIBSON, J. B. Oxford: Oxford University Press.

HOWELL, N. (1976) Toward a uniformitarian theory of human palaeodemography. In *The Demographic Evolution of Human Populations*, eds. WARD, R. H. and WEISS, K. M. London: Academic Press.

JALLE, O. R., COVE, W. R. and MCPHERSON, D. (1972) Population density and pathology: what are the relations for man. *Science. N.Y.*, **176**, 23–30.

JENNER, D., REYNOLDS, V. and HARRISON, G. A. (1979) Population field studies of catecholamines. In *Response to Stress*, ed. MACKAY, C. Guildford: IPC Science and Technology Press.

KETY, S. (1962) *Research Publications of the Association for Research in Nervous and Mental Disease*, vol. 40.

LADER, M. (1975) The nature of clinical anxiety in modern society. In *Stress and Anxiety*, eds. SPIELBERGER, C. D. and SARASON, I. G. New York: John Wiley & Sons.

LEIGHTON, A. H., LAMBO, T. A., HUGHES, C. C., LEIGHTON, D. C., MURPHY, J. M. and MACKLIN, D. B. (1963a) *Psychiatric Disorder among the Yoruba*. New York: Cornell University Press.

LEIGHTON, D. C., HARDING, J. S., MACKLIN, D. B., MACMILLAN, A. M. and LEIGHTON, A. H. (1963b) *The Character of Danger: Psychiatric Symptoms in Selected Communities*. New York: Basic Books.

LEVI, L. (1964) The stress of everyday work as reflected in productiveness, subjective feeling and urinary output of adrenaline and noradrenaline under salaried and piece-work conditions. *Journal of Psychosomatic Research*, **8**, 199–202.

LEVY, L. and ROWITZ, L. (1973) *The Ecology of Mental Disorders*. New York: Behavioural Publications.

LOGAN, W. P. D. and CUSHION, R. A. (1958) *Morbidity Statistics from General Practice*, Vol. 1. General Register Office. Studies on Medical and Population Subjects, No. 14. London: H.M.S.O.

LUNDBERG, U. (1976) Urban commuting: crowdedness and catecholamine excretion. *Journal of Human Stress.* **2,** 26 32.

MASON, J. W. (1959) Psychological influences on the pituitary–adrenal cortical system. *Recent Progress in Hormone Research.* **15,** 345–389.

MASON, J. W. (1972) Organization of psychoendocrine mechanisms: A review and reconsideration of research, In *Handbook of Psychophysiology*, eds. GREENFIELD, N. S. and STERNBACK, R. A. New York: Holt, Rinehart & Winston.

MCKEOWN, T. and LOWE, C. R. (1977) *An Introduction to Social Medicine.* Oxford: Blackwell Scientific Publications.

METZ, B., SCHAFF, G. and GRIVEL, F. (1960) Psychophysiological effects of sleep loss. *16th International Congress of Psychology Symposium on sleep loss.* Bonn.

MILLAR, S. E. (1976) Health and high density living in Hong Kong, Ph.D. Thesis, Australian National University.

MILLS, I. H. and EDEN, M. E. (1976) Social disturbances affecting young people in modern society. In *Man in Urban Environments*, eds. HARRISON, G. A., and GIBSON, J. B. Oxford: Oxford University Press.

NEEL, J. V. and WEISS, K. M. (1975) The genetic structure of a tribal population, the Yanomama Indians. *American Journal of Physical Anthropology*, **42,** 25–52.

OATES, J. (1974) *People in Cities.* Open University Press.

PERSKY, H., HAMBURG, D. A., BASOWITZ, H., GRINTER, R., SALSKIN, S., HARZ, M., BOARD, F. A. and HEATH, H. (1958) Relation of emotional responses and changes in plasma hydrocortisone level after stressful interviews. *Archives of Neurology and Psychiatry*, Chicago, **79,** 434–447.

POLITZER, W. M. and TUCKER, B. (1958). Urinary 17-ketosteroid and 17-ketogenic steroid excretion in South African Bantu. *Lancet*, 778–779.

REISEMAN, D. (1950) *The Lonely Crowd.* Garden City, New York: Anchor Books.

ROSE, G. A. (1976) Epidemiological evidence for the effects of the urban environment. In *Man in Urban Environments*, eds. HARRISON, G. A. and GIBSON, J. B. Oxford: Oxford University Press.

RUBEN, R. T., GUNDERSON, E. K. E. and ARTHUR, R. G. (1971) Life stress and illness patterns in the U.S. Navy. *Journal of Psychosomatic Research*, **15,** 89.

RUTTER, M. (1973) Why are London children so disturbed? *Proceedings of the Royal Society of Medicine*, **66,** 1221–1225.

SALKIND, M. R. (1973) The construction and validation of a self-rating anxiety inventory. Ph.D. Dissertation. University of London, reported in LADER, M. (1975) *loc. cit.*

SHAW, C. R. and MACKAY, H. D. (1942) *Juvenile Delinquency in Urban Areas.* Chicago: University of Chicago Press.

SIMPSON, H. W. (1967) Field studies of human stress in Polar regions. *British medical Journal*, **i,** 530–533.

SROLE, L., LANGNER, J. S., MICHAEL, S. T., OPLER, M. K. and RENNIE, T. A. C. (1962) *Mental Health in the Metropolis. The Midtown Manhattan Study.* New York: McGraw Hill.

TAYLOR, S. J. L. and CHAVE, S. (1964) *Mental health and environment.* London: Longmans.

TOLSON, W. W., MASON, J. W., SACKAR, E. J., HAMBURG, D. A., HANDLON, J. H. and FISHMAN, J. R. (1965) Urinary catecholamine responses associated with hospital admission in normal human subjects. *Journal of Psychosomatic Research*, **8,** 365–372.

WALLIS, C. P. and MALIPHANT, R. (1967) Delinquent areas in the county of London: ecological factors. *British Journal of Criminology*, **7,** 250–284.

WEINER, J. S. (1977) In *Human Biology*, eds. HARRISON, G. A., WEINER, J. S., TANNER, J. M. and BARNICOT, N. A. 2nd edn. Oxford: Oxford University Press.
WEST, D. J. (1973) *Who Becomes Delinquent?* London: Heinemann.
WING, J. K. (1974) Housing environments and mental health. In *Population and its Problems*, ed. PARRY, H. B. Oxford: Clarendon Press.
WING, J. K. (1976) Mental health. In *Man in Urban Environments*, eds. HARRISON, G. A. and GIBSON, J. B. Oxford: Oxford University Press.

THE ECOLOGY OF CHRONIC LUNG DISEASE

C. H. STUART-HARRIS

Department of Virology, University of Sheffield

THE chronic lung diseases of man form a group of apparently unrelated conditions affecting large numbers of persons over long periods of time and contributing significantly to mortality. The variation in mortality from one country to another of some components of the group was a major factor in arousing attention in the 1950s, largely because such differences suggested the causative importance of environmental factors. Nevertheless, until comparatively recently in developed and developing countries, pulmonary tuberculosis dominated the scene and it was the growing control over this disease which opened the way for research on causative factors in other chronic lung diseases.

The Major Forms of Chronic Lung Disease

The disorders listed in Table 1, adapted from Higgins's review of the epidemiology of chronic respiratory disease (1974), show important differences as well as resemblances between the UK and the USA. The table lists the mortality in 1967 as total numbers in three groups of conditions — pulmonary tuberculosis, cancer of the lung and chronic respiratory disease. Forming the latter are the three conditions of chronic bronchitis, emphysema and asthma, often bracketed as chronic non-specific lung disease (CNSLD) to indicate the lack of specificity of their causation, and pulmonary fibrosis, including occupational lung disease (pneumoconiosis). The numbers for

TABLE 1. Deaths and percentage distribution of respiratory disease United States and United Kingdom, 1967.

Cause of death	United States		United Kingdom	
	Number of deaths	% distribution	Number of deaths	% distribution
All causes	1 851 323	100·0	542 516	100·0
Chronic respiratory disease				
Asthma	4 137	0·2	1 757	0·3
Chronic non-specific lung disease { Bronchitis (chronic unqualified)	5 306	0·3	25 887	4·7
Emphysema	20 875	1·1	1 225	0·2
Pneumoconiosis	1 640	0·1	566	0·1
Other chronic interstitial pneumonia	4 219	0·2	467	0·1
Bronchiectasis	1 476	0·1	1 177	0·2
Other	2 790	0·2	279	0·1
Total	40 443	2·2	31 358	5·8
Cancer of trachea, lung and bronchus	54 407	2·9	28 252	5·2
Tuberculosis (respiratory)	6 351	0·3	1 798	0·3

(After Higgins, 1974.)

chronic non-specific lung disease illustrate a major difficulty of making international comparisons from mortality statistics. In the USA, the commonest component of CNSLD is emphysema, deaths from which at one time appeared to be increasing at an alarming rate but are now falling again. In the UK, on the other hand, chronic bronchitis has long been the leading cause of death, matching in total that from cancer of the lung. A visit to the UK early in the 1960s by a group of distinguished American doctors convinced them that British chronic bronchitis was a common American condition also, even though it did not appear on death certificates. It is now accepted that the apparent Anglo–American differences in mortality from these two different diagnostic conditions are semantic. The majority of patients with chronic bronchitis also exhibit emphysema and vice versa. Undoubted examples of each condition on its own do occur in both countries, but they form opposite ends of the spectrum, with a combination together of chronic bronchitis and emphysema as the large middle section. Nevertheless, semantic problems apart, there are still differences between the mortality from the total of CNSLD in Britain and the USA.

Table 2 shows the similar mortality statistics of 1974 comparing the USA with England and Wales, which has roughly one-quarter the total population of the former. That the totals for CNSLD in the two countries should be about the same indicates that there are about four

TABLE 2.   1974 deaths from selected causes of chronic lung diseases USA and England and Wales. From *Vital Statistics of the United States, 1974*, Vol. II. *Mortality*, Part A. US Department of Health, Education and Welfare, National Center for Health Statistics, Rockville, Maryland, and from *England and Wales, 1974. Mortality Statistics.* Series DH2. No. 1. H.M.S.O.

Cause of death	ICD no.	USA	England and Wales
Bronchitis, chronic and unqualified	490 – 1	5 097	24 089
Emphysema	492	19 907	1 423
Asthma	493	1 876	1 086
Total CNSLD	490 – 3	26 880*	26 598
Tuberculosis, respiratory	010 – 2	2 775	773
Cancer, respiratory	160 – 3	83 475	34 358

* A further 14 299 deaths in the USA were classified under 519–3 — chronic obstructive pulmonary disease. Total CNSLD (USA): 41 179.

times as many deaths proportionately in England and Wales than in the USA. Cancer of the lung also shows an excess in England and Wales, although this is only about half as great as the excess of deaths from CNSLD. These findings contrast with the relatively close resemblance between the deaths from pulmonary tuberculosis in the two countries.

Although death certificates furnish a dubious basis for international comparisons, they are valid within a particular country for comparing groups with different characteristics. Goodman, Lane and Rampling (1953) showed that there were considerable differences in bronchitis death-rates in different regions of England and Wales, which they attributed to the effects of urbanization. They also pinpointed the striking gradient in mortality between the different social classes I to V, based as these are upon occupations. The very high rates of the Standard Mortality Ratios for labourers and other

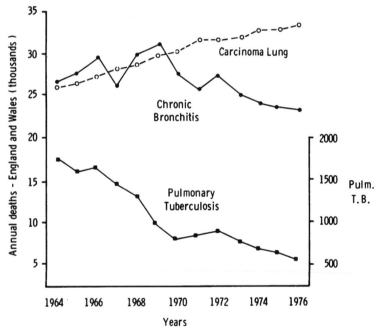

FIG. 1.   Data on mortality from chronic lung disease in England and Wales between 1964 and 1976. From *Mortality Statistics England and Wales, 1976*. Series DH2, No. 1. London: H.M.S.O.

unskilled workers in class V do not apply to those working in agriculture and this suggests the possible adverse effects of exposure to dust or smoke-polluted environments. Finally, mortality statistics indicate the age and sex variation in Britain, the rise in deaths with age being seen in both sexes above the age of 39. The male predominance (four- to five-fold) in those aged 45–64 is less at ages over 65. Inevitably, one must end this discussion of mortality statistics by enquiring about their validity. Trends and changes occurring with the passage of time are confirmatory. Fig. 1 shows the trends in gross numbers of deaths in England and Wales from 1964 to 1976 from three conditions—cancer of the lung, chronic bronchitis and pulmonary tuberculosis. Only the latter shows a considerable and favourable trend resulting from control over infection by the tubercle bacillus. Cancer of the lung, whose diagnosis in life can be made with certainty, continues to increase in gross numbers of deaths, but this is chiefly due to an increase among the older age-groups and also in women. The mortality from chronic bronchitis underwent an increase in the late 1960s coincidentally with two sharp influenza epidemics but is now decreasing. It is not possible to state whether this is a cohort effect or one of genuine decline due to the control of atmospheric pollution in the past 20 years. Finally, mortality statistics require to be validated through precise estimations of morbidity and this was the nub of the problem of chronic non-specific lung disease when enquiries began in 1950.

The Methodology of Investigation of CNSLD

The hunt for clues to the aetiology of chronic lung disease turns first of all on precise ascertainment of the prevalence of identifiable disease and then on a correlation of this with personal, familial and environmental factors. Pulmonary tuberculosis may be quoted as an example. There is no doubt concerning the recognition of infected persons or of the fact that there is no tuberculosis without the tubercle bacillus. Studies of groups of persons and of the course of the disease have, over the years, uncovered a complex interplay of personal factors such as nutrition, hormones and probably a genetic constitution of susceptibility. Environment also plays a part—witness the rise in mortality during influenza epidemics and the importance of social conditions.

Cancer of the lung is similarly readily identified in life and the graded relationship between cigarette smoking as a major causative factor was uncovered by studies of which the medical profession has cause to be proud. Yet Stocks (1959) suggested that regional and urban–rural differences in incidence could best be explained on the basis of exposure to pollution in towns. Whether or not this is related to carcinogenic constituents has not been established with certainty. There remains the third major component of chronic lung disease—chronic non-specific lung disease. Clinicians' diagnoses have been most in difficulty in the early stages of the long drawn-out struggle of chronic bronchitis, with its partial recovery from acute exacerbations and its steady downhill course once airways obstruction has appeared. Oswald's study on hospital patients carried out in 1953 (Oswald, Harold and Martin, 1953) showed that it was possible to suggest causative factors such as respiratory infections, the family, smoking and weather, but these might merely represent aggravating rather than initiating factors. Progess has depended upon the development of survey methods applicable to the community and the enunciation of definitions to replace diagnostic criteria. The Ciba Guest Symposium (1959) played a major role in the framing of definitions but the work of the Medical Research Council's Committee on the Aetiology of Bronchitis (Report, 1965) stimulated epidemiological enquiries needed to provide morbidity data. Respiratory symptoms elucidated by questionnaire and the measurement of pulmonary function in contrasting communities have afforded the basis of these studies. By this means, the existence of chronic productive cough on which the definition of chronic bronchitis is based, was measured. The disablement from airways obstruction, largely irreversible in nature and measured by relatively simple ventilatory tests, has substituted an objective measure for the subjective experience of breathlessness. These survey methods have now been adopted in many countries all over the world and have been endorsed by WHO (*Epidemiology of Chronic Non-specific Respiratory Diseases*, 1957).

Of the two other components of CNSLD, emphysema has so far defied epidemiological study in life, largely because of the difficulty of its differentiation from generalized airways obstruction. Its definition in pathological terms, and by measurement of alveolar wall interfaces, has led to comparisons of thin lung slices from autopsies mounted on paper. Thurlbeck, Ryder and Sternby (1974) have thus compared the prevalence in necropsy material in three cities — Montreal, Malmöe and Cardiff. Hope arose fifteen years ago that emphysema would prove to be largely a genetic disorder due to deficiency of serum α1-antitrypsin, but since then it has been shown that it is only the homozygous person who is chiefly at risk (Kueppers, Briscoe and Bearn, 1964; Kueppers, Fallat and Larson, 1969; Lieberman, 1969). Asthma has thus far defied an all-embracing definition useful for epidemiological work. This is largely because reversal of acute airways obstruction originally used to define asthma requires pharmacological methods. The clinician is less inhibited. He recognizes and has partial understanding at least of juvenile asthma with its faulty allergic constitution and link with eczema. Yet its immunological abnormality renders its victims subject to the vicissitudes of infection, inhalation of foreign proteins and occasional termination in death. But the intrinsic asthma of middle life is less readily distinguished from chronic bronchitis, for the obstruction of the airways does not yield readily to treatment and is relatively less influenced by the environment.

Epidemiological Studies on Chronic Bronchitis with Airways Obstruction

Much has now been learnt concerning the ecology of this condition. The questionnaire drawn up through the MRC Committee concentrates upon questions, tested for their reliability and low error, in relation to cough, sputum and chest illnesses. Ventilatory tests need to be simple, highly reproducible and gaining ready co-operation from those who are being surveyed. Table 3 shows the basic methods. Enquiry concerning breathlessness has not been so rewarding as measurement of the FEV. The complaint of wheezing has, surprisingly enough, proved useful in relation to disablement. The exclusion of localized lung disease by radiological methods is necessary when dealing with communities in which a high incidence has occurred of pulmonary tuberculosis. Bronchograms cannot be used in the field and so bronchiectasis has to be grouped with bronchitis with which, in fact, it often co-exists.

Thus the prevalence of chronic bronchitis and of generalized airways obstruction can be measured in contrasting groups and communities. The once-for-all prevalence study is improved by

TABLE 3.   Methodology of epidemiological studies of chronic non-specific lung
disease (Chronic Bronchitis. Emphysema and Asthma)

Questionnaire		
Key Questions	Cough—Morning	
	Winter	
	Three months per year	
	Sputum—Morning	
	Winter	
	Three months per year	
	Chest illnesses—Past 3 years	
	Three weeks or more	
Pulmonary function tests		
Forced expiratory volume (1 second)		$FEV_{1.0}$
Forced vital capacity		FCV
Ratio FEV/FVC		
Peak flow rate		PFR
Flow-volume curves		MMEF rate

repetition at a later date or in a systematic prospective manner, as
shown by Fletcher and his colleagues (Fletcher et al. 1976). The choice
of contrasting groups is the key to learning the interplay of personal
and environmental factors, which will now be discussed.

Ecological Factors in Chronic Bronchitis with Airways Obstruction

Cigarette smoking

Each and every field study made in Britain, the USA and elsewhere
has shown the great importance of cigarette smoking in relation to the
incidence of chronic bronchitis. Table 4 shows the influence of
smoking on prevalence in the rural population aged 55 to 64 of
Annandale (Dumfriesshire) studied by Higgins and Cochran (1958)
compared with industrial men at Staveley (Derbyshire) in two age-
groups (Higgins et al, 1959).

The relationship is not only that between symptoms and smoking
or an absence of smoking, for there is also a graded relationship
between the consumption of cigarettes and incidence of bronchitis as
in the case of carcinoma of the lung. Fletcher et al. (1970) also found a
graded relationship between smoking and the mean annual decline of
the FEV in a group of working men in London with early chronic
bronchitis studied annually. Thurlbeck, Ryder and Sternby (1974)
found a similar correlation between the degree of emphysema of the
lungs at autopsy in the cities of Montreal, Cardiff and Malmö and

TABLE 4. Influence of smoking on respiratory symptoms in a rural (Annandale) and an urban area (Staveley). (After Higgins and Cochrane, 1958, and Higgins *et al.*, 1959.)

Population and age-group	Smoking category and number	Respiratory symptoms			
		Cough sputum	Chest illness	Breathless ness	Chronic bronchitis
Annandale 55–64	Non-smoker (6)	0	0	2 (33·3%)	0
	Ex-smoker (13)	1 (7·7%)	5 (38·5%)	3 (23·1%)	1 (7·7%)
	≤ 14/day (38)	6 (15·8%)	6 (15·8%)	10 (26·3%)	2 (5·3%)
	≥ 15/day (37)	12 (32·4%)	6 (16·2%)	12 (32·4%)	3 (8·1%)
Staveley 25–34	Non-smoker (56)	5 (8·9%)	4 (7·1%)	3 (5·4%)	2 (3·6%)
	Ex-smoker (31)	4 (12·9%)	7 (22·6%)	0	4 (12·9%)
	≤ 14/day (193)	43 (22·3%)	25 (13%)	17 (8·8%)	13 (6·7%)
	≥ 15 day (89)	39 (43·8%)	11 (12·4%)	11 (12·4%)	7 (7·9%)
Staveley 55–64	Non-smoker (29)	1 (3·4%)	2 (6·9%)	5 (17·2%)	1 (3·4%)
	Ex-smoker (62)	13 (21%)	13 (21%)	20 (32·3%)	8 (12·9%)
	≤ 14/day (157)	61 (38·9%)	41 (26·1%)	63 (40·1%)	32 (20·3%)
	≥ 15/day (136)	70 (51·5%)	39 (28·7%)	62 (45·6%)	30 (22·1%)

personal smoking habits in life. Smokers had an average emphysema score 3- to 10-fold that of non-smokers. Clearly smoking is a major factor in both chronic bronchitis and emphysema and one which can overshadow all others. It probably accounts for the observed differences in bronchitis prevalence between men and women.

Yet smoking cannot be held to account for all the differences observed in international comparisons and particularly those between men of like age and occupation. The first of these international studies was a comparison of symptoms and the FEV in men living on the Danish island of Bornholm with other groups studied by the MRC Pneumoconiosis Unit. Olsen and Gilson (1960) compared men from the town of Rønne with those living in agricultural areas of Britain whose tobacco consumption was much higher. Lower rates of respiratory symptoms and a higher FEV were found in the Danish men, a greater proportion of whom were non-smokers. Holland *et al.*, (1965) carried out an Anglo-American study in 1960–61 on van drivers in the telephone branch of the Post Office in London and three English country towns with outside telephone workers in three areas of the USA. Apart from an increased prevalence of the symptoms of CNSLD in British men compared with Americans of like age, the

TABLE 5. The pulmonary function ($FEV_{1.0}$) of postal and outside telephone workers in England and Wales and the USA graded by smoking habits and standardized for age 40. (After Holland. 1966.)

Smoking habits	London		English country towns		USA towns	
	No.	Mean $FEV_{1.0}$	No.	Mean $FEV_{1.0}$	No.	Mean $FEV_{1.0}$
Non-smoker	13	3·0	30	3·1	89	3·7
Ex-smoker	36	2·8	77	3·0	89	3·7
Smokers						
1–14 G/day	74	2·7	142	3·0	60	3·6
15–24 G/day	98	2·7	134	2·9	169	3·4
25+ G/day	29	2·5	40	2·9	218	3·4
Total	250	2·7	423	3·0	625	3·5

findings relating to the FEV were of considerable interest. Table 5 shows that in both populations, whose ages were from 40 to 59, there was an inverse graded relationship between cigarette smoking and the mean FEV. In both non-smokers and smokers of similar numbers of cigarettes, the mean FEVs in British men were lower than those of the American men. This finding was thought to suggest the effect of exposure of British men to higher levels of atmospheric pollution, perhaps for many years.

Atmospheric pollution

Ever since the disastrous London smog in December 1952 when 4000 excess deaths occurred during and after a four-day intensely polluted fog, it has been clear that a combination of high concentrations of smoke particles and SO_2 can be lethal to persons suffering from chronic bronchitis and emphysema. Even lesser pollution episodes in London (Waller and Lawther, 1955) and Sheffield (Clifton *et al.*, 1960) caused increased symptoms, a rise in sickness incapacity and even temporarily increased mortality of those already suffering from chronic bronchitis. With the reduction in smoke followed by a later decrease in atmospheric SO_2 which followed the Clean Air Act, there has been a notable absence of acute rises in pollution during foggy weather and the effects in exacerbating symptoms can no longer be observed (Lawther, Waller and Henderson, 1970).

Atmospheric pollution of a lesser but chronic variety does, however, impose a hazard from birth onwards. This is apparent in comparative studies on urban and rural communities such as that made nationally by the British College of General Practitioners (1961). In this study, residence, smoking habits and social class appeared to be concerned in the higher rates of CNSLD associated with urban life. Much more important has been the demonstration of the harmful effects of pollution in early childhood. Here cigarette smoking has not yet begun, but as Douglas and Waller (1966) showed by a cohort study of 5000 children born in 1946 throughout Britain, a higher rate of acute lower respiratory tract illnesses such as bronchitis and pneumonia was experienced during the first five years of life by those children living in the most polluted areas, judged by coal consumption.

Colley, Douglas and Reid (1973) followed up 3899 of these same children when they were adults of 20. Those with a history of chest illness before the age of 2 and who were exposed to heavy air pollution in childhood, had a greater prevalence of chronic cough than those without this childhood history, whether or not they had become cigarette smokers (Table 6). Colley and Reid (1970) further studied 10 000 children aged 6 to 10 living in contrasting rural areas of England and Wales. There was a pronounced paternal social class gradient in the frequency of chronic cough and a history of bronchitis in the children. But only children from parents of Social Classes 4 and 5 showed the effect of exposure to increasing levels of air pollution by a pronounced urban–rural gradient. Thus the effect noted so long ago by Goodman, Lane and Rampling (1953) in contrasts in mortality is

TABLE 6. % prevalence of cough, day or night in winter (adults aged 20 years). (After Colley, Douglas and Reid 1973.)

History of smoking	Chest illness under 2 year	Air pollution grade in childhood (coal consumption and years of exposure)			
		Light (7 – 17)		Heavy (18 – 28)	
		Social class father		Social class father	
		1 + 2	3 + 4	1 + 2	3 + 4
Never	None	4·7 (344)	5·7 (369)	4·7 (277)	6·6 (212)
	One or more	12·3 (57)	8·3 (108)	8·3 (84)	10·8 (102)
Present	None	11·2 (214)	12·6 (325)	14·1 (192)	15·7 (261)
Cigarette Smokers	One or more	16·4 (55)	11·8 (102)	12·3 (73)	22·2 (144)

confirmed by a study of symptoms in young children. Moreover, the fact that the child is father to the man is not only applicable in Britain.

Burrows, Knudson and Lebowitz (1977) studied young adults living in Tucson in Arizona and showed that among comparable cigarette smokers, a history of chronic respiratory disease in childhood including asthma was related to an increased prevalence of chronic cough and sputum in adult life.

Such studies now point strongly to the seeds of CNSLD being formed in childhood when social class and urban dwelling combine with greater frequency of episodes of acute infection. It is, of course, impossible to rule out a genetic predisposition to chronic respiratory disease and the effect of the family will be discussed below.

Infection

The role of infection by bacteria, *mycoplasma* and viruses in relation to chronic bronchitis has been repeatedly surveyed. (Leeder, 1975; Stuart-Harris 1965, 1968; Tager and Speizer, 1975) and cannot be repeated here. A chronic bacterial colonization of the airways by *Haemophilus influenzae* and *Streptococcus pneumoniae* is a feature of the middle and later stages of CNSLD, but it not so readily discernible in earlier phases. Acute viral infections punctuate both earlier and later stages (Stenhouse, 1967, 1968; Fisher *et al.*, 1969) but are only followed by an exacerbation of symptoms in a proportion of instances.

The recent findings of the effect on the pulmonary function of healthy persons of simple acute respiratory virus infections, particularly if they are cigarette smokers (Fridy *et al.*, 1974), is of great importance. As such infections are repetitive throughout life, it is clear that they may be significant in determining the gradual decline with age in the ventilatory function and even the development of airways obstruction. Leeder, Gill and Peat (1974) found that influenza virus infection of adult men and women caused a reduction in the maximal mid-expiratory flow rate suggestive of mild airways obstruction even during convalescence. Influenza virus attenuated in virulence for healthy persons can sometimes cause acute exacerbation of symptoms and increased airways obstruction in patients with chronic bronchitis (Winson *et al.*, 1977). Acute attacks of asthma in children also appear to be precipitated by rhinovirus infections (Minor *et al.*, 1974). Thus it is easy to see why respiratory virus infections can be associated with acute illnesses or even death in those with previous chronic disease.

What is yet to be discovered is the role of infection in the initiation of chronic disease and this probably requires that more studies should be made in childhood with a follow-up into adult life. It is possible that studies in developing countries may give a lead in this connection.

The effects of climate and environment

In European countries, patients with CNSLD suffer acute exacerbations of their symptoms particularly during winter-times. There is also a seasonal rise in mortality at such times. Infections due to respiratory viruses play some role in connection with this, but cold, damp weather and particularly fog unquestionably exert an unfavourable effect. Burrows and Lebowitz (1975) state that the warm dry climate of Arizona, to which large numbers of patients with asthma and emphysema flock, is associated with a less regular seasonal exacerbation of symptoms and drier cough.

Studies made by Australian workers in New Guinea on communities (Woolcock and Blackburn, 1967; Anderson, 1974, 1976) have shown that chronic non-tuberculous lung disease is common in these islanders. Woolcock, *et al.* (1970) describe this disease as chronic bronchitis and emphysema together with extensive fibrosis of the lungs and pleura. The latter could reflect repeated acute respiratory infections said to be common in children. Smoke pollution of native huts, smoking of home-grown tobacco early in adolescence (Anderson, 1974) and overcrowding in the communal huts all appear to be causative factors which are not so very different from those of European civilizations.

The methodology of such studies in primitive people involves a change from that of questionnaire. Anderson (1976), who found that asthma was rare in the New Guinea Highlands, used a physical sign—the loose cough sign—previously suggested by Hall and Gandevia (1971) as an alternative to questions concerning daily sputum. It is obvious that much more work requires to be carried out on the best approach to the investigation of chronic lung disease in developing countries. Nevertheless, cigarette smoking is world-wide and its insidious effect can be based on childhood habits in the tropics as in temperate zones (Elegbeleye and Femi-Pearse, 1976). There is evidence from the West Indies and Guyana (Miller 1974) that black races of Africa origin are less susceptible to the effects of smoking on the airways than Indian or white races.

Occupation

Though frequently claimed as a major factor in the incidence of chronic bronchitis, occupation has proved to be an elusive subject. Beginning with the view that dusty non-siliceous atmospheres are the reason for the high rates of mortality in foundry-workers and miners, a major setback was the discovery that the wives of both sets of workers also exhibit an excess mortality compared with wives of men with less hazardous occupations. A most careful set of studies carried out by Lowe and his colleagues on steel-workers in South Wales showed that there was little evidence that exposure to airborne dust was as important a factor as cigarette smoking (Lowe, 1969; Lowe *et al.*, 1968; Lowe, Campbell and Khosla, 1970). In fact, cigarette smoking and social factors are major obstacles to the discernment of the effect of occupation alone. The very high rates of sickness absence in coal miners in the UK from bronchitis is hard to evaluate because absences from most other causes of sickness are also higher than in other workers. Nevertheless, the study of the prevalence of chronic bronchitis in miners and non-miners living in the same district (Higgins *et al.*, 1956) consistently shows a higher rate in miners.

Exposure to siliceous dust has, of course, long been accepted as the cause of pulmonary fibrosis and pneumoconiosis in steel fettlers, coal-workers, sandblasters and many other exposed groups. Yet it transpires that there is no doubt that chronic bronchitis with airways obstruction in persons with pneumoconiosis is responsible for much of the disability. Even gold-miners who are exposed to air with a higher siliceous content than that of coal-miners appear to exhibit higher rates of chronic bronchitis than non-miners even after allowing for the effects of age and smoking (Sluis-Cremer, Walters and Sichel, 1967).

Finally, vegetable dusts cause respiratory symptoms and even airways obstruction probably through a different mechanism. The byssinosis of cotton-workers is not confined to Lancashire (Schilling, 1956) but occurs in cotton ginnery workers in the Sudan (Khogali, 1976) and in Egypt and the USA. The pharmacological effects of cotton dust extracts (Bouhuys, Lindell and Lundin, 1960; Nicholls,

1962) seem more likely to be the reason for constriction of the muscle of the bronchi on Monday mornings than an hypothetical allergic action. Even so the productive cough in these workers may be due to an irritant action on the bronchi akin to that of chronic bronchitis.

Familial background

At the end of the nine-year prospective study of chronic bronchitis of London transport workers, Fletcher *et al.* (1976) concluded that there is a personal factor which renders some persons particularly susceptible to the harmful effects of smoking and air pollution. They deduced this largely from the variable rates of decline of the FEV in different persons, which appear to be relatively independent from the symptoms of chronic bronchitis alone. They were not able to define this susceptibility, yet it agrees with the suggestive evidence of a familial factor in chronic bronchitis.

Hints at the likelihood of familial involvement in chronic bronchitis were obtained early in the 1960s by a comparison of the histories of bronchitis in sisters and wives of persons with or without chronic bronchitis in Sheffield (Stuart-Harris, 1964). An elegant study by Kueppers *et al.* (1977) confirms earlier observations that the frequency of chronic obstructive pulmonary disease in the siblings of patients with this disorder is twice or thrice the rate in siblings of other matched control subjects. Measurements of the $FEV_{1.0}$ indicated a higher rate of airways obstruction in the relatives of patients with chronic bronchitis not explained by cigarette consumption. These authors suggested that heterozygosity of α1-antitrypsin deficiency could be the predisposing factor in the relatives, but admit that other genetic or environmental factors are probably concerned. This contrasts with the negative results of the community studies of obstructive lung disease and protease-inhibitor phenotypes reported by Morse *et al.* (1977). One cannot forget also that children share together the same family environment, the same risk of respiratory infections and exposure to polluted air while they are young and such factors may be equally as important as the genetic constitution.

Conclusions

Semantic differences make international comparisons of individual conditions such as chronic bronchitis and emphysema of relatively little use but it is clear that total deaths from chronic non-specific lung disease (CNSLD) are excessive in Britain. Prevalence studies in different communities living in different areas and of persons in the same or in different occupations, show that it is probable that both environmental and personal factors are concerned in the aetiology of chronic obstructive bronchitis. Cigarette smoking is the most important causative factor in relation to symptoms (sputum), to airways obstruction, and to emphysema at post-mortem. Air pollution from smoke and sulphur dioxide is regarded as an important factor in the frequency of lower respiratory tract infections in infants and children. It is also responsible for exacerbations of illness in adults with established chronic bronchitis, and severe pollution episodes cause increased numbers of deaths in such persons. Infections of the respiratory tract by both bacteria and viruses appear to cause illnesses sometimes accompanied by changes in the pulmonary function in both normal persons and those with existing chronic lung disease. They may initiate chronic disease in children living in adverse environments which may render them more vulnerable to the harmful effects of smoking in later (adult) life.

Social factors and occupation also exert an influence on chronic lung disease although their actions are difficult to disentangle from those of the above-mentioned causes. Personal factors of a genetic character (α-antitrypsin deficiency) appear to be responsible for a small proportion of cases of emphysema. A familial susceptibility also exists in the case of chronic bronchitis, but this may either be genetic or attributable to adverse environment in early childhood.

References

ANDERSON, H. R. (1974) Smoking habits and their relationship to chronic lung disease in tropical environment in Papua New Guinea. *Bulletin de Physio-Pathologie Respiratoire*, **10**, 619–633.

ANDERSON, H. R. (1976) Respiratory abnormalities and ventilatory capacity in a Papua New Guinea Island Community. *American Review of Respiratory Diseases*, **114**, 537–548.

BOUHUYS, A., LINDELL, S.-E. and LUNDIN, G. (1960) Experimental studies on byssinosis. *British Medical Journal*, **1**, 324–326.

BURROWS, B. and LEBOWITZ, M. D. (1975). Characteristics of chronic bronchitis in a warm, dry, region. *American Review of Respiratory Diseases*, **112**, 365–370.

BURROWS, B., KNUDSON, R. J. and LEBOWITZ, M. D. (1977). The relationship of childhood respiratory illness to adult obstructive airways disease. *American Review of Respiratory Diseases*, **115**, 751–760.

CIBA GUEST SYMPOSIUM (1959) Terminology, definitions and classification of chronic pulmonary emphysema and related conditions. *Thorax*, **14**, 286–299.
CLIFTON, M., KERRIDGE, D., PEMBERTON, J., MOULDS, W. and DONOGHUE, J. K. (1960) Morbidity and mortality from bronchitis in Sheffield in four periods of severe air pollution. *Proceedings of the International Conference on Clean Air*, 1959, pp. 189–192.
COLLEGE OF GENERAL PRACTITIONERS (1961) Chronic bronchitis in Great Britain. *British Medical Journal*, **2**, 973–979.
COLLEY, J. R. T. and REID, D. D. (1970) Urban and social origins of childhood bronchitis in England and Wales. *British Medical Journal*, **2**, 213–217.
COLLEY, J. R. T., DOUGLAS, J. W. B. and REID, D. D. (1973) Respiratory disease in young adults: influence of early childhood lower respiratory tract illness, social class, air pollution and smoking. *British Medical Journal*, **3**, 195–198.
DOUGLAS, J. W. B. and WALLER, R. E. (1966) Air pollution and respiratory infection in children. *British Journal of Preventive and Social Medicine*, **20**, 1–8.
ELEGBELEYE, O. O. and FEMI-PEARSE, D. (1976) Incidence and variables contributing to onset of cigarette smoking among secondary schoolchildren and medical students in Lagos, Nigeria. *British Journal of Preventive and Social Medicine*, **30**, 66–70.
EPIDEMIOLOGY OF CHRONIC NON-SPECIFIC RESPIRATORY DISEASES (1975) *Bulletin of the World Health Organization*, **52**, 251–260.
FISHER, M., AKHTAR, A. J., CALDER, M. A., MOFFAT, M. A. J., STEWART, S. M., ZEALLEY, H. and CROFTON, J. W. (1969) Pilot study of factors associated with exacerbations of chronic bronchitis. *British Medical Journal*, **4**, 187–192.
FLETCHER, C. M., PETO, R., SPEIZER, F. S., and TINKER, C. M. (1970) A follow-up study of the natural history of obstructive bronchitis. In *Bronchitis III*, pp. 103–116. International Symposium at Gröningen, The Netherlands, Eds. ORIE, N. G. M. and VAN DER LENDE, Assen: Royal Van Gorum.
FLETCHER, C., PETO, R., TINKER, C. and SPEIZER, F. E. (1976) *The Natural History of Chronic Bronchitis and Emphysema*. Oxford: Oxford University Press.
FRIDY, W. W., JR., INGRAM, R. H., HIERHOLZER, J. C. and COLEMAN, M. T. (1974) Airways function during mild viral respiratory illnesses. The effect of rhinovirus infection in cigarette smokers. *Annals of Internal Medicine*, **80**, 150–155.
GOODMAN, N., LANE, R. E. and RAMPLING, S. B. (1953) Chronic bronchitis: an introductory examination of existing data. *British Medical Journal*, **2**, 237–243.
HALL, G. J. L. and GANDEVIA, B. (1971) Relationship of the loose cough sign to daily sputum volume. *British Journal of Preventive and Social Medicine*, **25**, 109–113.
HIGGINS, I. T. T. (1974) *Epidemiology of Chronic Respiratory Diseases: a Literature Review*. Washington, D.C. 20460: Office of research and development, Environmental Protection Agency.
HIGGINS, I. T. and COCHRAN, J. B. (1958) Respiratory symptoms, bronchitis and disability in a random sample of an agricultural community in Dumfriesshire. *Tubercle*, **39**, 296–301.
HIGGINS, I. T. T., COCHRANE, A. L., GILSON, J. C. and WOOD, C. H. (1959) Population studies of chronic respiratory disease. Comparison of miners, foundry-workers and others in Staveley. *British Journal of Industrial Medicine*, **16**, 255–268.
HIGGINS, I. T. T., OLDHAM, P. D., COCHRANE, A. L. and GILSON, J. L. (1956) Respiratory symptoms and pulmonary disability in an industrial town. *British Medical Journal*, **2**, 904–909.
HOLLAND, W. W. (1966) The study of geographic differences in the prevalence of chronic bronchitis. *The Statistician*, **16**, 5–22.
HOLLAND, W. W. REID, D. D., SELTSER, R. and STONE, R. W. (1965) Respiratory disease in England and the United States. *Archives of Environmental Health*, **10**, 338–343.

KHOGALI, M. (1976) Byssinosis: a follow-up study of cotton ginnery workers in the Sudan. *British Journal of Industrial Medicine*, 33, 166–174.

KUEPPERS, F., BRISCOE, W. A. and G. (1964) Hereditary deficiency of serum alpha-1-antitrypsin. *Science*, 146, 1678–1679.

KUEPPERS, F., FALLAT, R. and LARSON, R. K. (1969) Obstructive lung disease and alpha-1-antitrypsin deficiency gene heterozygosity. *Science*, 165, 899–901.

KUEPPERS, F., MILLER, R. D., GORDON, H., HEPPER, N. G., and OFFORD, K. (1977) Familial prevalence of chronic obstructive pulmonary disease in a matched pair study. *American Journal of Medicine*, 63, 336–342.

LAWTHER, P. J. WALLER, R. E. and HENDERSON, M. (1970) Air pollution and exacerbations of bronchitis. *Thorax*, 25, 525–539.

LEEDER, S. R. (1975) Role of infection in the cause and course of chronic bronchitis. *Journal of Infectious Diseases*, 131, 731–742.

LEEDER, S. R., GILL, P. W. and PEAT, J. K. (1974). Short and long-term effects of influenza A on lung function. *Medical Journal of Australia*, 2, 812–814.

LIEBERMAN, J. (1969) Heterozygous and homozygous alpha-1-antitrypsin deficiency in patients with pulmonary emphysema. *New England Journal of Medicine*, 281, 279–284.

LOWE, C. R. (1969) Industrial bronchitis. *British Medical Journal*, 1, 463–468.

LOWE, C. R., CAMPBELL, H. and KHOSLA, T. (1970) Bronchitis in two integrated steelworks. 3. Respiratory symptoms and ventilatory capacity related to atmospheric pollution. *British Journal of Industrial Medicine*, 27, 121–129.

LOWE, C. R., PELMEAR, P. L., CAMPBELL, H., HITCHENS, R. A. N., KHOSLA, T. and KING, T. C. (1968) Bronchitis in two integrated steelworks 1. Ventilatory capacity, age and physique of non-bronchitic men. *British Journal of Preventive and Social Medicine*, 22, 1–11.

MILLER, G. J., (1974) Cigarette smoking and irreversible airways obstruction in the West Indies. *Thorax*, 29, 495–504.

MINOR, T. E., DICK, E. C., DeMEO, A. N., OUELLETTE, J. J., COHEN, M. and REED, C. E. (1974) Viruses as precipitants of asthmatic attacks in childhood. *Journal of the American Medical Association*, 227, 292–298.

MORSE, J. O., LEBOWITZ, M. D., KNUDSON, R. J. and BURROWS, B. (1977) Relation of protease-inhibitor phenotypes to obstructive lung disease in a community. *New England Journal of Medicine*, 296, 1190–1194.

NICHOLLS, P. J. (1962) Some pharmacological actions of cotton dust and other experimental dusts. *British Journal of Industrial Medicine*, 19, 33–41.

OLSEN, H. C. and GILSON, J. C. (1960) Respiratory symptoms, bronchitis and ventilatory capacity in men. An Anglo-Danish comparison. *British Medical Journal*, 1, 450–456.

OSWALD, N. C., HAROLD, J. T. and MARTIN, W. J. (1953) Clinical pattern of chronic bronchitis. *Lancet*, ii, 639–643.

REPORT TO THE MRC by the Committee on the Aetiology of Chronic Bronchitis (1965) Definition and classification of chronic bronchitis for clinical and epidemiological purposes. *Lancet*, i, 775–779.

SCHILLING, R. S. F. (1956) Byssinosis in cotton and other textile workers. *Lancet*, ii, 261–265, 319–325.

SLUIS-CREMER, G. K., WALTERS, L. G. and SICHEL, H. S. (1967) Chronic bronchitis in miners and non-miners: an epidemiological survey in a community in the gold-mining area in the Transvaal. *British Journal Industrial Medicine*, 24, 1–12.

STENHOUSE, A. C. (1967) Rhinovirus infection in acute exacerbations of chronic bronchitis: a controlled prospective study. *British Medical Journal*, 3, 461–463.

STENHOUSE, A. C. (1968) Viral antibody levels and clinical status in acute exacerbations of chronic bronchitis: a controlled prospective study. *British Medical Journal*, **3**, 287 290.

STOCKS, P. (1959) Cancer and bronchitis mortality in relation to atmospheric pollution and smoke. *British Medical Journal*, **1**, 74 79.

STUART-HARRIS, C. H. (1964) Discussion on heredity of bronchitis. In *Bronchitis II*, pp. 29–31. International Symposium at Groningen, The Netherlands, Eds. ORIE, N. G. M. and SLUITER, H. J., Assen, Royal Van Gorcum.

STUART-HARRIS, C. H. (1965) The role of infection in chronic bronchitis. *Medicina Thoracalis*, **22**, 39–47.

STUART-HARRIS, C. H. (1968) The role of bacterial and viral infection in chronic bronchitis. *Archives of Environmental Health*, **16**, 586–595.

TAGER, I. and SPEIZER, F. E. (1975) Role of infection in chronic bronchitis. *New England Journal of Medicine*, **292**, 563–571.

THURLBECK, W. M., RYDER, R. C. and STERNBY, N. (1974) A comparative study of the severity of emphysema in necropsy populations in three different countries. *American Review of Respiratory Diseases*, **109**, 239–248.

WALLER, R. E. and LAWTHER, P. J. (1955). Some observations on London fog. *British Medical Journal*, **2**, 1356–1358.

WINSON, I. G., SMIT, J. M., POTTER, C. W. and HOWARD, P. (1977) Studies with live attenuated influenza virus in chronic bronchitis. *Thorax*, **32**, 726–728.

WOOLCOCK, A. J. and BLACKBURN, C. R. B. (1967) Chronic lung disease in the territory of Papua and New Guinea—an epidemiological study. *Australian Annals of Medicine*, **16**, 11–19.

WOOLCOCK, A. J., BLACKBURN, C. R. B., FREEMAN, M. H., ZYLSTRA, W. and SPRING, S. R. (1970) Studies of chronic (non-tuberculous) lung disease in New Guinea populations. *American Review of Respiratory Diseases*, **102**, 575–590.

ECOLOGICAL FACTORS IN MULTIPLE SCLEROSIS IN NORTH-EAST SCOTLAND

DAVID I. SHEPHERD

Department of Neurology, North Manchester General Hospital,
Crumpsall, Manchester

and ALLAN W. DOWNIE

Department of Medicine, Aberdeen University, Aberdeen

MULTIPLE sclerosis (M.S.) is at the same time one of the more unpleasant and one of the most fascinating chronic disorders of the central nervous system; unpleasant because it can and does, although not inevitably, cause disablement even among young adults; fascinating because of the many tantalizing clues which hint at, but do not prove its cause.

Definition

Before a disease can be surveyed, criteria of diagnosis must first be established and this is more difficult in M.S. than in most diseases, as there is no test, laboratory or clinical, which gives conclusive proof of the diagnosis. While patchy loss of myelin around nerve fibres within the central nervous system is regarded as strong pathological evidence for the disease, this is not available in life and diagnosis depends on deductions drawn from the clinical story plus the findings on examination. The results of some laboratory tests may support the diagnosis but in the end, certainty of diagnosis is expressed only as a degree of probability, e.g. 'probable', 'early probable and latent', or 'possible' M.S. While most experienced neurologists would agree about the diagnosis in a majority of situations, a number of patients labelled 'possible' M.S. might give cause for dispute. The occurrence of episodes of involvement of the central nervous system, disseminated in place and time, would strengthen the diagnosis but neither automatically confirms it, nor indeed is essential to it, in some patients in whom other supportive laboratory evidence may be present. Difficulties in ascertainment and assessment of borderline cases could partly explain the variation in prevalence rates noted in different parts of the world, were it not for the fact that medical specialism in the more prosperous countries has developed in parallel fashion with similar standards in, and free communication between them.

Epidemiological studies in the larger less well developed countries at one time were necessarily scanty and falsely low levels of prevalence rate there might have been partly explained on this basis. Increasing standards of general and medical care in many of these countries has not, however, led to a major change in prevalence figures and the unique geographical variations recognized for some years still hold, even though repeated studies of restricted populations often produce some evidence of apparently increasing prevalence. This may be in part artifactual.

World-wide Distribution

It has been found that this disease in essence is rare in tropical countries and increases in prevalence with increasing latitude (Barlow, 1966). Prevalence rates for tropical countries are under 5 per 100 000 of the population. For Northern Europe, including England, rates vary between 50 and 100 per 100 000 (Shepherd, 1976). Northeast Scotland is even higher at 140 per 100 000 (Shepherd, 1976), and the Orkney Isles (300 per 100 000) and the Shetlands have the highest prevalence in the world (Poskanzer et al., 1976). This pattern of variation with latitude is not entirely consistent, however; Japan, for instance, having a much lower prevalence rate (2 to 4 per 100 000) (Kuroiwa and Shibasaki, 1976) than might be expected. Associated with variations in latitude are many climatic, geophysical and biological variables which might require consideration as aetiologic factors. Differing susceptibilities because of particular racial factors also might explain geographical variation and here there is already much suggestive evidence. Certain tissue types akin to blood groups, designated the HLA groups, can be determined and it is now clearly evident that certain HLA antigens are over-represented in patients with M.S. (Compston *et al.*, 1978) and may occur with varying frequency in different racial groups. This probably means that people with these tissue types are more susceptible to M.S. than those without, but does not mean that having one of these tissue types automatically causes or indeed is essential for the development of M.S. Studies in migrants show too that the possible harmful factor related to residence in a temperate country may be countermanded by migration at an early age to a tropical climate (Dean and Kurtzke, 1971). Evidence for the opposite effect is as yet uncertain. It is said that no single case of M.S. has been found in the population of 11 000 000 South African Bantu (Dean, 1967), yet M.S. is recognized as not rare in North American Negroes of African extraction (Leibowitz and Alter, 1973). This might suggest that the protective factor accorded to race or to residence in a tropical country might be reduced by migration to a country of temperate climate and higher prevalence.

The relative importance of the genetic, as opposed to some acquired, factor in this change of prevalence still requires elucidation. Migration studies also suggest that people emigrating in childhood from a high to a low prevalence area acquire the prevalence of the country to which they emigrate. Those emigrating after the age of 15 carry a prevalence rate closer to their country of birth (Dean and Kurtzke, 1971). Such fluctuations suggest the possibility of a childhood infective factor in the causation of M.S. and there has been much work suggesting possible relationships with common viruses for instance, measles (Johnson and Nelson, 1977); some work suggesting a relationship with less common viruses e.g., canine distemper (Cook and Dowling, 1978), and some speculation about the possibility of unknown 'slow' viruses (Fraser, 1977). Earlier implication of other forms of bacterial infection seems to have been disproved. It seems likely that if a common virus is to be implicated, the subsequent development of M.S. would have to depend on an unusual immunologic response. A combination of an external environmental factor, possibly viral with an unusual immunologic response which might, in turn, be linked to genetic factors associated with the possession of particular tissue types, would indeed help to make sense of the apparently conflicting strands of evidence as regards the aetiology of this condition. The concept of multifactorial causation of disease is fashionable, although not new. The possibility that there is a single determining factor of prime aetiologic importance still exists. However, until this can be confirmed, further studies along various lines of research will still be needed, including careful epidemiological studies. These can, with advantage, be carried out in the United Kindom where prevalence is relatively high, communications good and standards of medical care and record keeping above average. In addition to these factors, in north-east Scotland, all patients suspected of having M.S. are liable to be referred to a single medical centre for evaluation. For these reasons, therefore, we have studied the occurrence of M.S. in north-east Scotland and certain ecological factors affecting its distribution.

North-east Scotland

We have carried out two point prevalence studies of M.S. in northeast Scotland. The area comprised the City of Aberdeen and counties of Aberdeen, Kincardine, Moray and Banff which is almost equivalent to the Grampian Region. We used the 1971 Census population for both studies (General Register Office, 1974). The prevalence of M.S. on 1 December 1970 was 127 cases per 100 000 population and on 1 December 1973 it was 144 cases per 100 000 (Table 1). The 1973 prevalence rate is the highest recorded in any surveyed area of comparable population. The only higher figures are from the Orkney and Shetland surveys, with a population of less than 35 000 (Fog and Hyllested 1966; Poskanzer et al., 1976), and two small communities of under 5000 population in the USA (Deacon et al., 1959; Koch et al., 1974).

TABLE 1.   Prevalence of multiple sclerosis in north-east Scotland by sex in 1970 and 1973.

	Number	Prevalence per 100 000 population*
1970 Study		
All patients	557	127
All men	215	102
All women	342	149
1973 Study		
All patients	634	144
All men	232	110
All women	402	175

* Population in 1971 (General Register Office 1974) was 440 176: men 210 250; women 229 926.

Age and sex

Women are affected by M.S. more frequently than men and usually in the ratio 3 : 2, as we found in north-east Scotland (Table 1). Since the disease is rare before the age of 20 and after 70, age and sex specific prevalence rates more accurately reflect its frequency. In the 1973 study, adapting the 1971 census data (General Register Office, 1974), the highest age specific prevalence rate for men was 282 per 100 000 population for those aged 50–59 and for women 384 per 100 000 population for those aged 40–49 (Fig. 1). Indeed among the 104 000 people aged 40 to 59 in north-east Scotland, one in every 306 had M.S.; a rate higher than any previously reported.

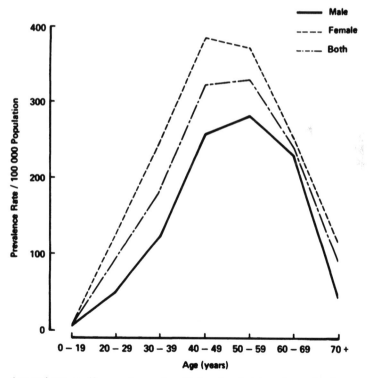

Age and sex specific prevalence of multiple sclerosis in north-east Scotland on 1 December 1973. Based on the age and sex distribution of the whole Scottish population in census 1971 (General Register Office, 1974).

Geographical variation

For our studies, we divided north-east Scotland into 28 geographical units based on administrative districts, but combining adjacent districts where necessary to produce unit populations of over 10 000. The prevalence rates on 1 December 1970, for areas in which people were living, ranged from 46 per 100 000 to 251 per 100 000 population and showed a highly significant deviation from a random distribution (Shepherd and Downie, 1978). No significant distribution was found for area of birthplace using the same geographical units, but the same area unit had the greatest prevalence rate for both area of birthplace and area of residence in 1970. If environmental factors are important in the aetiology of M.S., then in this area unit they have been operating for many years.

In north-east Scotland, Aberdeen is the only major city and the rest of the region is largely rural. The prevalence rate for the City of Aberdeen for area of residence in 1970 did not differ significantly from the rest of the region. For area of birthplace, fewer cases than expected were recorded for Aberdeen City, but the deficit was not significant compared with the rest of north-east Scotland. This study, and more definitely those in Northern Ireland (Ashitey and Millar, 1970) and in Finland (Wikström, Myllylä and Kivalo, 1972), suggest that the risk of developing M.S. is less for those born in large urban centres. Other studies, however, have shown either no urban–rural difference (Poskanzer, Schapira and Miller, 1963) or suggested an excess urban risk (Beebe *et al.*, 1967).

Clustering

The presence of time–space clustering in a disease suggests a possible "infective" aetiology. The most spectacular M.S. cluster involved four out of seven research workers who developed the disease having previously worked intensively with the disease swayback in lambs (Campbell *et al.*, 1947).

Subsequently, no reasonable explanation has been established for this puzzling group of cases. It is even more puzzling when one considers that swayback itself is considered to be linked with copper deficiency and is not thought to have an infective aetiology. Campbell *et al.* (1950) also reported six patients with M.S. all living within the same small village. Millar (1966) described two high risk areas in Northern Ireland; one containing seven patients in a population of

1000 and the other seven in a population of 500. In the only formal statistical analysis involving M.S. patients, however, no evidence of clustering was found by the methods used (Ashitey and MacKenzie, 1970; Hargreaves and Merrington, 1973). In north-east Scotland, we found two instances of the type of clustering already described. One involved two adjacent parishes in the geographical unit with the highest prevalence rate in the 1970 study. In 1970 one in 380 people in these parishes (population 2650 in 1971 census) had M.S., but in the previous 40 years, a total of 21 patients had lived in the area for varying periods, twelve being the maximum number in any single year. The other instance involved an isolated valley in which no patients were living in 1970 or 1973, but where seven patients were born between 1913 and 1930. During this period 291 children were born and survived at least 1 year and of these 1 in 70 boys and 1 in 30 girls later developed M.S. (Shepherd, 1976). This cluster emphasizes the value of studying birthplace of patients rather than current address. Probably these are chance findings, but the statistical significance could be tested by either the space–time analysis of Knox (1964) or preferably the case-control method of Pike and Smith (1974).

Monthly and seasonal occurrence of onset or exacerbation
    Limburg (1950) suggested that because of the association of M.S. with colder climates, a seasonal occurrence of onset or exacerbation might occur, but neither he nor others (Hopkins and Swank, 1955; Schapira, 1959; Thygesen 1953) could demonstrate it. Wüthrich and Rieder (1970), however, found a minimum incidence in the autumn and a significant excess of attacks in the first half of the year. Attacks of optic neuritis occurred more commonly between April and July (Bradley and Whitty, 1967; Taub and Rucker, 1954), but a statistically significant excess was found only by Hutchinson (1976). In north-east Scotland, the exact month of occurrence of 116 episodes of optic neuritis in 112 patients was known (Table 2). Only a marginally significant difference in the number of episodes by month was found, but again most attacks occurred between April and July, with another peak in October. The seasonal distribution also showed no significant difference from that expected using the method of David and Newell (1965). More recently, Compston *et al.* (1978) have suggested that the season of occurrence of optic neuritis may have prognostic value with

TABLE 2. Month of occurrence of episodes of optic neuritis in north-east Scotland.

Month	No. of episodes	Month	No. of episodes
January	9	July	10
February	9	August	4
March	9	September	4
April	9	October	17
May	11	November	9
June	18	December	7
	65		51

d.f. = 11, χ^2 = 20·55, $P < 0·05$.

respect to future development of M.S. Thus onset of optic neuritis was more common in summer (54 per cent) than winter but of the latter, 48 per cent went on to develop M.S. as compared to 31 per cent of the former. This suggested the possibility of at least two forms of optic neuritis with different aetiologies.

Occupation and socio-economic classification
Interest has long existed in the possible association of M.S. and particular occupations (Bramwell, 1917) and social class. Miller, Ridley and Schapira (1960) found a significant excess of social classes I and II among men in Northumberland and Durham based on occupation at onset of M.S. A similar distribution by social class was found in Oxford (Russell, 1971). In north-east Scotland we found a marked excess of social class I and a moderate excess of social class III among economically active men at onset of M.S. (Shepherd, 1976). The Registrar General's Decennial Supplements for England and Wales (1938, 1958, 1971) contain information on the social class status of M.S. patients. No consistent pattern emerges, but this is not surprising, since analysis was by social class at the time of death rather than onset. A chronic disorder like M.S. inevitably leads to downgrading in social class status and the greater risk postulated for higher social classes would be minimized by analysis at the time of death.

Russell (1971) also analysed his men by 'collapsed socio-economic groups' (Office of Population, Censuses and Surveys, 1973) and found a significant excess of employers managers, farmers and professional workers. We found, however, a significant excess of only professional

workers at the 2 per cent level. Economically active women in north-east Scotland had a marked excess of socio-economic groups 5 and 6 (clerical workers, shop assistants, teachers and nurses) (Shepherd, 1976).
Half a century ago, agricultural workers, carpenters and woodworkers were thought to have an excess occupational risk of M.S. (Dreyfuss, 1921; McAlpine 1927), but control population information was lacking. In contrast, Sutherland and Wilson (1951) were unable to find any vulnerable occupation among 173 men in Glasgow. North-east Scotland provided a unique opportunity of comparing the occupations of all known M.S. patients with accurate occupational information from the whole population (General Register Office, 1966). Among woodworkers there was a highly significant excess of M.S. patients (Swinscow, 1976) and this was even more striking among joiners and carpenters alone (Shepherd, 1976). One in every 258 joiners and carpenters had M.S. compared with 1 in 632 of the male working population of north-east Scotland. Similarly, among doctors, 1 in 143 had M.S., but although significant, the number affected was small. Among the economically active women with M.S., 12·9 per cent were nurses compared with an expected 5·4 per cent. Thus one in 200 nurses had M.S. and this figure excludes several women with onset prior to starting nursing, whilst engaged in other occupations.

Familial and conjugal multiple sclerosis
    Relatives of M.S. patients have the disease more often than the general population. The frequency of familial M.S. varies widely in different prevalence surveys (Table 3), but it seems to increase as the overall prevalence rate increases. This alone, however, could not explain the varied geographical prevalence. First-degree relatives are affected more often than distant relatives and the rate for affected siblings is greater than that for affected parents (Table 4). In north-east Scotland the difference was less marked than in other studies. Mackay and Myrianthopoulos (1966) found an exceptional sibling rate, but they were trying to find the concordance rate of M.S. in twins and their mode of selection was by public appeal for 'twins with multiple sclerosis'. This biased selection undoubtedly contributed to the high sibling rate. They did find a higher concordance rate for monozygotic (23·1 per cent) than dizygotic twins (20·7 per cent).

TABLE 3. Familial occurrence of multiple sclerosis in different surveys.

Reference	Survey area	No. of families	% with more than one affected member
Thygesen (1953)	Denmark	60	16·7
Allison (1963)	Orkney and Shetländ	60	11·7
Study (1973)	North-east Scotland	614	9·8
Gudmundsson (1971)	Iceland	88	9·1
Millar and Allison (1954)	Northern Ireland	668	6·6
Schapira et al. (1963)	North-east England	607	5·8
Kuroiwa et al. (1975)	Japan	1084	2·0
Alter et al. (1962)	Israel	282	0

TABLE 4. Frequency of affected siblings and parents in different surveys.

Reference	Survey area	Affected siblings		Affected parents	
		Number	%	Number	%
Mackay and Myrianthopoulos (1966)	USA	14/236	5·9	2/115	1·7
Study (1973)	North-east Scotland	30/2109	1·4	15/1250	1·2
Millar and Allison (1954)	Northern Ireland	34/2939	1·2	11/1336	0·8
Schapira et al. (1963)	North-east England	21/2151	1·0	9/1206	0·8

Among cousins, these authors found 0·4 per cent who had M.S., which is higher than the general population rate, but lower than that of siblings and parents.

Conjugal M.S. is rare and only 30 instances had been reported up to 1975 (Shepherd, 1976), but in three of these a child was affected as well. The rate of conjugal M.S. probably does not exceed the prevalence rate of M.S. in the general population.

HLA antigens

A definite association between M.S. and certain HLA antigens has become evident in recent years. The initial association was with HLA-A3 and HLA-B7, but more recently, stronger associations have been noted with the D locus antigen HLA-Dw2 (formerly LD-7a) and a B lymphocyte alloantigen now provisionally named HLA-DRw2 (Batchelor, Compston and McDonald, 1978). These associations hold true for north Europeans, but different associations have emerged for other ethnic groups. The world-wide occurrence of HLA-B7 shows a pattern similar to the distribution of M.S., and this antigen has been found in a higher percentage of a control population from north-east Scotland than in any other control series (Shepherd and Downie, 1978). This may imply that a larger reservoir of potential patients exists in north-east Scotland than elsewhere, but it is not the sole factor contributing to the high prevalence rate.

Conclusions

We have identified several ecological factors of importance in the aetiology and distribution of M.S. in north-east Scotland. Women, particularly in certain age groups, are more prone to the disease. The region constitutes a high risk zone throughout which the risk is not spread homogeneously. Firm evidence of clustering would support the presence of an environmental factor, but the examples given require valid statistical appraisal. The varied seasonal and monthly occurrence is of interest and again implies an environmental factor. Higher social class or socio-economic status clearly carries a greater risk of development of M.S., but is there a real occupational risk? Further supportive evidence is required, but for joiners, and carpenters it would appear so. For doctors and nurses increased exposure may be a relevant factor, deserving further investigation.

There is a familial M.S. risk, but is this genetically or environmentally determined? In support of a genetic origin is the increasing frequency of familial M.S. in ascending order through cousins, parents, siblings, dizygotic to monozygotic twins, thus suggesting a recessive pattern of inheritance. Against recessive inheritance are the facts that the concordance rate in monozygotic twins is lower than it should be, there is no excess of affected children of conjugal M.S. parents and there is not an increased parental consanguinity rate (Shepherd, 1976). Support for an environmental aetiology comes from the fact that affected siblings and parents have been in close contact for prolonged periods and exposed to the same exogenous agents, but then one would expect an increased conjugal rate. In our studies, in 16 out of 69 families the affected members had never met and in a further 13 instances contact was minimal. On balance, the increased familial occurrence of M.S. provides stronger evidence of a genetic than of an environmental factor and this is also suggested by the definite HLA associations. Almost certainly both factors are involved in the aetiology and as Morris (1975) said "more than the spirochaete is involved in primary syphilis". We are left with the question, does M.S. occur more frequently in north-east Scotland than elsewhere? We think this is unlikely. North-east Scotland is a compact geographical unit with a largely stable population. It affords an ideal situation for epidemiological study with the likelihood of almost complete case ascertainment. Of more convincing importance, however, the mortality rate for M.S. in north-east Scotland does not exceed the overall Scottish rate (Annual Reports, Registar General, 1939–1974; Shepherd, 1976). Multiple sclerosis, therefore, is probably common throughout Scotland.

References

ALLISON, R. S. (1963) Some neurological aspects of medical geography. *Proceedings of the Royal Society of Medicine*, **56**, 71–76.

ALTER, M., HALPERN, L., KURLAND, L. T., BORNSTEIN, B., LEIBOWITZ, U. and SILBERSTEIN, J. (1962) Multiple sclerosis in Israel. Prevalence among immigrants and native inhabitants. *Archives of Neurology*, **7**, 253–263.

Annual Reports of the Registrar-General for Scotland (1939–1974) Edinburgh: H.M.S.O.

ASHITEY, G. A. and MACKENZIE, G. (1970) 'Clustering' of multiple sclerosis cases by date and place of birth. *British Journal of Preventive and Social Medicine*, **24**, 163–168.

ASHITEY, G. A. and MILLAR, J. H. D. (1970) Multiple sclerosis in Northern Ireland; a study of the date and place of birth of patients. *Ulster Medical Journal*, **39**, 55–63.

BARLOW, J. S. (1966) Solar-flare induced increases in sea level cosmic ray intensities and other geophysical phenomena in relation to multiple sclerosis. *Acta Neurologica Scandinavica*, **42**, suppl. 19, 118–136.

BATCHELOR, J. R., COMPSTON, D. A. S. and McDONALD, W. I. (1978) The significance of the association between HLA and multiple sclerosis. *British Medical Bulletin*, **34**, 279–284.

BEEBE, G. W., KURTZKE, J. F., KURLAND, L. T., AUTH, T. L. and NAGLER, B. (1967) Studies on the natural history of multiple sclerosis. *Neurology*, **17**, 1–17.

BRADLEY, W. G. and WHITTY, C. W. M. (1967) Acute optic neuritis: its clinical features and their relation to prognosis for recovery of vision. *Journal of Neurology, Neurosurgery and Psychiatry*, **30**, 531–538.

BRAMWELL, B. (1917) Etiology of disseminated sclerosis. *Edinburgh Medical Journal*, **18**, 96–106.

CAMPBELL, A. M. G., DANIEL, P., PORTER, R. J., RUSSELL, W. R., SMITH, H. V. and INNES, J. R. M. (1947) Disease of the nervous system occurring among research workers on swayback in lambs. *Brain*, **70**, 50–58.

CAMPBELL, A. M. G., HERDAN, G., TATLOW, W. F. T. and WHITTLE, E. G. (1950) Lead in relation to disseminated sclerosis. *Brain*, **73**, 52–71.

COMPSTON, D. A. S., BATCHELOR, J. R., EARL, C. J. and McDONALD, W. I. (1978) Factors influencing the risk of multiple sclerosis developing in patients with optic neuritis. *Brain*, **101**, 495–511.

Cook, S. D. and Dowling, P. C. (1978) Multiple sclerosis and canine distemper. *Lancet*, i, 605–606.

David, H. A. and Newell, D. J. (1965) The identification of annual peak periods for a disease. *Biometrics*, **21**, 645–650.

Deacon, W. E., Alexander, L., Siedler, H. and Kurland, L. T. (1959) Multiple sclerosis in a small New England community. *New England Journal of Medicine*, **261**, 1059–1061.

Dean, G. (1967) Annual incidence, prevalence, and mortality of multiple sclerosis in white South-African-born and in white immigrants to South Africa. *British Medical Journal*, **2**, 724–730.

Dean, G. and Kurtzke, J. F. (1971) On the risk of multiple sclerosis according to age at immigration to South Africa. *British Medical Journal*, **3**, 725–729.

Dreyfuss, H., (1921) Multiple Sklerose und Beruf. *Zeitschrift für die Gesamte Neurologie und Psychiatrie*, **73**, 479–507.

Fog, M. and Hyllested, K. (1966) Shetland–Orkney–Faroe project. *Acta Neurologica Scandinavica*, **42**, suppl. 19, 6–11.

Fraser, K. B. (1977) Multiple sclerosis: A virus disease? *British Medical Bulletin*, **33**, 34–39.

General Register Office (1966) *Census 1961 Scotland, Occupation and Industry*, County Tables, Aberdeen City and Counties of Banff, Kincardine, Moray, Nairn and Aberdeen. Edinburgh: H.M.S.O.

General Register Office (1974) *Census 1971 Scotland, Population Tables*. Edinburgh: H.M.S.O.

Gudmundsson, K. R. (1971) Clinical studies of multiple sclerosis in Iceland. A follow-up of previous study and reappraisal. *Acta Neurologica Scandinivica*, **47**, suppl. 48, 5–78.

Hargreaves, E. and Merrington, M. (1973) A note on the absence of clustering of multiple sclerosis cases. *Journal of Chronic Diseases*, **26**, 47–50.

Hopkins, C. and Swank, R. (1955) Multiple sclerosis and the local weather. *Archives of Neurology and Psychiatry*, **74**, 203–207.

Hutchinson, W. M. (1976) Acute optic neuritis and the prognosis for multiple sclerosis. *Journal of Neurology, Neurosurgery and Psychiatry*, **39**, 283–289.

Johnson, K. P. and Nelson, B. J. (1977) Diagnostic usefulness of cerebrospinal fluid in clinical neurology. *Annals of Neurology*, **2**, 425–431.

Knox, E. G. (1964) Epidemiology of childhood leukaemia in Northumberland and Durham. *British Journal of Preventative and Social Medicine*, **18**, 17–24.

Koch, M. J., Reed, D., Stern, R. and Brody, J. A. (1974) Multiple sclerosis: A cluster in a small North-Western United States community. *Journal of the American Medical Association*, **228**, 1555–1557.

Kuroiwa, Y., Igata, I., Itahara, K., Koshijima, S., Tsubaki, T., Toyokura, Y. and Shibasaki, H. (1975) Nationwide survey of multiple sclerosis in Japan. *Neurology*, **25**, 845–851.

Kuroiwa, Y. and Shibasaki, H. (1976) Epidemiologic clinical studies of multiple sclerosis in Japan. *Neurology*, **26**, no. 6, Part 2, 8–10.

Leibowitz, U., and Alter, M. (1973) *Multiple Sclerosis, Clues to its Cause*, Amsterdam: North Holland/American Elsevier, p. 134.

Limburg, C. (1950) The geographic distribution of multiple sclerosis and its estimated prevalence in the United States. In *Multiple Sclerosis and the Demyelinating Diseases*, Association for Research into Nervous and Mental Disease Vol. 28, Baltimore: Williams and Wilkins Company. p. 15–24.

McAlpine, D. (1927) Disseminated sclerosis: with special reference to its infective origin. *British Medical Journal*, **1**, 269–273.

MACKAY, R. P. and MYRIANTHOPOULOS, N. C. (1966) Multiple sclerosis in twins and their relatives: final report. *Archives of Neurology*. **15**, 449–462.

MILLAR, J. H. D. (1966) Multiple sclerosis: two high risk areas in Northern Ireland. *The Journal of the Irish Medical Association*, **59**, 138–143.

MILLAR, J. H. D. and ALLISON, R. S. (1954) Familial incidence of disseminated sclerosis in Northern Island, *Ulster Medical Journal*, **23**, suppl. 2, 29–92.

MILLER, H., RIDLEY, A. and SCHAPIRA, K. (1960) Multiple sclerosis, a note on social incidence. *British Medical Journal*, **2**, 343–345.

MORRIS, J. N. (1975) *Uses of Epidemiology*. 3rd Ed., Edinburgh: Churchill Livingstone. p. 174.

OFFICE OF POPULATION, CENSUSES AND SURVEYS (1973) *General Household Survey* Social survey division, p. 61. London: H.M.S.O.

PIKE, M. C. and SMITH, P. G. (1974) A case-control approach to examine diseases for evidence of contagion, including diseases with long latent periods. *Biometrics*, **30**, 263–279.

POSKANZER, D. C., SCHAPIRA, K. and MILLER, H. (1963) Epidemiology of multiple sclerosis in the counties of Northumberland and Durham. *Journal of Neurology, Neurosurgery and Psychiatry*, **26**, 368–376.

POSKANZER, D. C., WALKER, A. M., YONKONDY, J. and SHERIDAN, J. L. (1976) Studies in the epidemiology of multiple sclerosis in the Orkney and Shetland Islands. *Neurology*, **26**, No. 6. Part 2. 14–17.

RUSSELL, W. R. (1971) Multiple sclerosis: occupation and social group at onset. *Lancet*. **ii**, 832–834.

SCHAPIRA, K. (1959) The seasonal incidence of onset and exacerbation in multiple sclerosis. *Journal of Neurology, Neurosurgery and Psychiatry*, **22**, 285–286.

SCHAPIRA, K., POZKANZER, D. C. and MILLER, H., (1963) Familial and conjugal multiple sclerosis. *Brain*, **86**, 315–332.

SHEPHERD, D. I. (1976) Multiple sclerosis in North-East Scotland, MD Thesis, University of Aberdeen.

SHEPHERD, D. I. and DOWNIE, A. W. (1978) Prevalence of multiple sclerosis in North-East Scotland. *British Medical Journal*, **2**, 314–316.

SUTHERLAND, J. M. and WILSON, D. R. (1951) Disseminated sclerosis in man and experimentation with sheep. *Glasgow Medical Journal*, **32**, 302–310.

SWINSCOW, T. D. V. (1976) Statistics at square one. IX Percentages. *British Medical Journal*, **2**, 166–167.

TAUB, R. G. and RUCKER, C. W. (1954) The relationship of retrobular neuritis to multiple sclerosis. *American Journal of Ophthalmology*. **37**, 494–497.

The Registrar-General's Decennial Supplement (1938) *England and Wales 1931*. Part IIa, Occupational mortality. London: H.M.S.O.

The Registrar-General's Decennial Supplement (1958) *England and Wales 1951*, Part II, Vol. 2, Occupational mortality. London: H.M.S.O.

The Registrar-General's Decennial Supplement (1971) *England and Wales 1961*. Occupational mortality Tables. London: H.M.S.O.

THYGESEN, P. (1953) *The Course of Disseminated Sclerosis. A Close-up of 105 Attacks*, p. 118. Copenhagen: Rosenkilde and Bagger.

WIKSTRÖM, J., MYLLYLÄ, G. and KIVALO, E. (1972) Studies on genetic factors in the epidemiology of multiple sclerosis in Finland. *Scandinavian Journal of Clinical and Laboratory Investigation*, **29**, suppl. 122. 80.

WÜTHRICH, R. and RIEDER, H. P. (1970) The seasonal incidence of multiple sclerosis in Switzerland. *European Neurology*, **3**, 257–264.

INTERNATIONAL AND URBAN-RURAL VARIATION IN CANCER

OLE M. JENSEN

International Agency for Research on Cancer, Unit of Epidemiology and Biostatistics

THE agglomeration of human beings into large urban societies leads to fundamental changes in nature's ecological system, of which humans form an integral part. The influences of urbanization on human biology were already intuitively realized by Hippocrates, who taught that the well-being of humans was related to environmental factors: seasons, winds, waters, places, vegetation and way of life.

Never before in his history has man lived through such fundamental and rapid changes of society as in the last few centuries, and it is pertinent to ask how he adapts to the parallel man-made modifications of his environment. Chronic disorders have assumed increasing importance after the successful fight against infectious diseases in the economically developed part of the world, and it has been suggested that the upsurge of a number of chronic diseases is associated with changes in the environment.

Epidemiological evaluation of such associations is made difficult by the lack of long-standing health statistics of comparable quality in many countries. The question may be approached by cross-sectional comparisons of populations with different degrees of affluence, but this is becoming increasingly difficult in the 'old' world because of the trend towards homogeneity. The epidemiologist may, therefore, resort to comparisons with developing parts of the world, keeping in mind the introduction of new variables, such as climatic, racial and cultural differences; it should be stressed that both the developed and developing parts of the world may benefit from such research into the causation of disease.

This paper deals with one aspect of the reaction of the human body—cancer—to economic development and urbanization as judged by the distribution of malignant diseases, both internationally and within nations.

Size of the Problem

Cancer as a public health problem

Knowledge of the frequency of cancer in various parts of the world has greatly improved during this century. Mortality in selected countries since 1950 has been published by Segi and Kurihara (1960–1972), and the World Health Organization publishes mortality statistics annually (World Health Organization, 1978).

Table 1 shows cancer deaths as a proportion of all deaths in selected countries of the five continents. Although there is a lack of information from the developing parts of Africa and Asia, the available data indicate that cancer, as a whole, is a public health problem in the developed parts of the world, contributing around 20 per cent of all deaths in North America, Europe, Australia and Japan. Developing countries of Africa, Asia and South America are still dominated by other health problems, cancer contributing only around 5 per cent of all deaths.

TABLE 1.   Cancer deaths in 1973 as a proportion (%) of all deaths in selected countries

Country	Males	Females
Africa	2·1–5·6	1·1–6·0
Egypt	2·1	1·1
Mauritius	5·6	6·0
America	1·7–20·5	3·8–21·6
Mexico	3·6	5·7
United States	17·7	18·5
Asia	2·6–22·4	2·5–20·0
Japan	20·0	18·5
Thailand	2·6	2·5
Europe	12·6–26·5	11·4–24·5
England and Wales	22·1	19·2
Italy	21·1	17·9
Poland	18·4	18·2
Oceania	17·7–18·6	17·7–19·0
Australia	17·7	17·7

These differences between the developed and the developing parts of the world are in part a reflection of different age-structures, with fewer persons surviving to cancer ages in Africa, Asia and South America. As a consequence, cancer becomes proportionately more important in the developed parts of the world as other causes of death, such as infections diseases — dominating in developing countries — are suppressed. Estimates of the size of the cancer problem, in absolute terms, can therefore only be based on morbidity or mortality rates.

Cancer morbidity

Morbidity from cancer has now been quantified in many parts of the world through the systematic compilation of data by national or regional Cancer Registries (Waterhouse *et al.*, 1976). Difficulties exist in comparing morbidity rates between different registries, particularly when comparisons are made between countries in different stages of development with regard to medical facilities (Doll, 1976), i.e., availability, quality and use of medical services. Some of the potential biases introduced by these difficulties are minimized by restricting comparisons to the age-range 35 to 64 (i.e., age-standardized, truncated rates) (Doll and Cook, 1967). This has been done in Fig. 1, which shows the cancer morbidity in selected countries and areas. In addition, Fig. 1 shows the cumulative incidence rates for the same countries, at ages 0 to 74, i.e., the approximate proportion of the population who would develop cancer before the age of 75 if no other causes of death were in operation (Day, 1976).

A 2- to 2·5-fold range in incidence is observed among both males and females. Although there is a regrettable abundance of blank areas on the world map of Cancer Registries in Africa, Asia and, to a certain extent, South America, it appears that cancer is almost as frequent in many of these places as in Europe and North America. Thus Chinese males in tropical Singapore have more cancer than men in Oxford, and there is only some 10% difference between Norway, Cali (Colombia) and Bombay (India). Among females, the highly developed USA and Japan take the highest and lowest positions, respectively; European, Asian, South American and African regions occupy intermediate positions.

The concept that cancer, in general, is exclusively a disease of the developed part of the world, closely associated with industrialization,

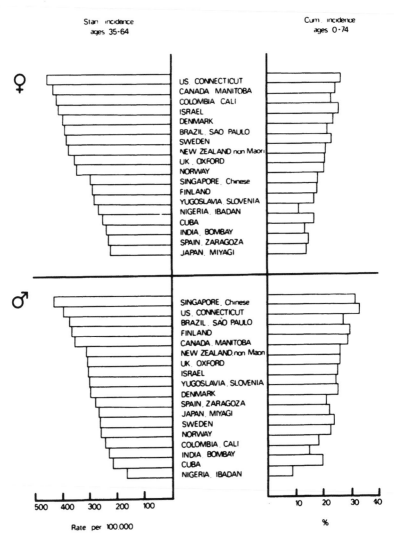

FIG. 1.   Age-standardized, truncated incidence rates (ages 35 to 64) and cumulative incidence rates (ages 0 to 74) of all cancers in selected countries.

should thus be abandoned. Some 15 to 25 per cent of the population develops cancer before the age of 74 irrespective of where in the world it lives (see Fig. 1).

International Variation in Cancer Patterns

The cancer patterns differ between different countries and societies. Examples from selected Cancer Registries are presented in Fig. 2, as the proportion of age-standardized incidence rates for the four most frequent cancers in any one region, out of all neoplasms registered (excluding skin cancers). The detailed three-digit code of the international classification of disease (World Health Organization, 1967) provides for 61 cancer sites. Fig. 2 shows that in any given country, and for either sex, only four different sites provide roughly 50 per cent of the total load of neoplasms; in Oxford (England) and Miyagi (Japan) approximately 45 per cent of all cancers among males are located to a single organ, lung and stomach, respectively.

The homogeneity of the cancer pattern in Europe and North America is striking. Among males, lung, stomach and prostate cancer predominates, and among females, breast, colon and stomach cancer. Occasional changes in this pattern, such as the high rectal cancer rate among Danish men (Jensen *et al.*, 1974) and the high incidence rate of larynx cancer among Spanish men in Zaragoza, provide interesting areas for aetiological research.

Although highly industrialized like Europe and North America, Japan shows a different cancer pattern, dominated by the high frequency of stomach cancer in both sexes (Fig. 2), and by low rates for large bowel cancer (Waterhouse *et al.*, 1976). High rates of stomach cancer are also observed among males in Colombia. The otherwise rare cancers of the naso-pharynx take fourth position among Singapore Chinese males, and the cancer pattern among Bombay men is dominated by cancers of the mouth, larynx and oesophagus.

A completely different distribution is seen in Ibadan Nigeria (Fig. 2), where primary liver cancer and malignant lymphomas (lymphosarcomas, Hodgkin's Disease) predominate among males. Ratio studies of cancer in other parts of Africa are consistent with these findings (Tuyns and Ravisse, 1970).

In line with observations in the developing countries of Asia and South America, the cervix uteri is the most frequent cancer site among

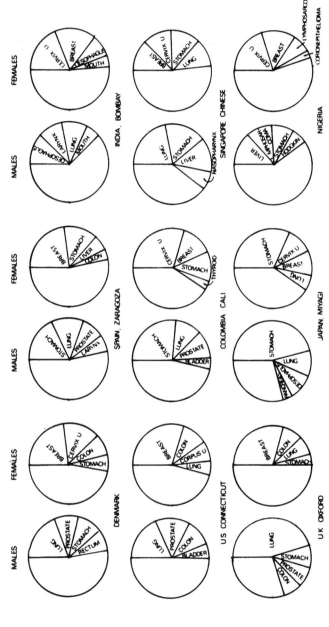

FIG. 2. Four most frequent cancers as proportion of all malignant neoplasms in selected countries.

women in Ibadan (Fig. 2). The high frequency of chorionepithelioma in Africa is also apparent from Fig. 2, bringing this tumour to fourth position in Ibadan women.

These examples of different patterns of cancer morbidity indicate that the international variation in the incidence of cancers at specific sites is, in general, much larger than the 2- to 2·5-fold difference observed for all cancers taken together (Fig. 1). Cancer of the oesophagus thus shows a more than 50-fold variation internationally (Doll, 1969) with 'hot-spots' in Iran across Asia to Northern China, among South African Bantus and in the Caribbean; the highest incidence of oesophageal cancer in Europe is seen in the north-west of France (Tuyns and Massé, 1975 a, b). Primary liver cancer is particularly frequent in Africa and Asia; a 5- to 10-fold difference exists for cancer of the colon, which is frequent in Europe and the United States, and lung cancer varies almost 15-fold internationally. Specific cancers are thus associated with specific environments, or factors present in a given setting, be it African, Indian or English. Such variation in cancer occurrence provides a tool for unravelling factors of aetiological importance, potentially enabling preventive regulations or measures to be introduced.

Urban–Rural Variation

Sources of error

The influence of urban life on cancer morbidity may be examined by relating mortality or morbidity rates to the degree of urbanization. Such comparisons undertaken within countries tend to minimize the sources of error affecting international comparisons, but differences in the availability, quality and use of medical services constitute nevertheless a general problem, which may bias the results. In addition, it is difficult to compare urban–rural ratios between countries, owing to varying definitions of the terms urban and rural, as discussed recently by Frederici *et al.* (1976).

Table 2, based on data from the Cancer Registry (Clemmesen, 1977), exemplifies the difficulties encountered even in Denmark, where they may be taken to be minimal in the rather small, homogeneous population with a high standard of living reaching all strata of the population, and with a highly developed social security system and good medical care. Easy access to medical facilities is confirmed by the fact that approximately the same proportion of

TABLE 2. Verification of diagnosis of selected cancers 1968–1972 in Copenhagen and Danish rural districts (%) (from Clemmesen, 1977)

Site	Area	Males				Females			
		Diagn. in hosp.	Histol. verified	Deaths autopsied	Known by death cert. only	Diagn. in hosp.	Histol. verified	Deaths autopsied	Known by death cert. only
Oesophagus	Copenhagen	99	92	80	1·2	93	78	66	6·9
	Rural	91	73	37	9·0	91	75	37	8·6
Colon	Copenhagen	99	90	78	0·6	98	88	70	2·2
	Rural	95	75	35	5·0	90	72	33	9·9
Lung	Copenhagen	95	81	87	4·6	97	80	86	2·8
	Rural	94	71	48	6·2	92	60	49	8·5
Breast	Copenhagen	96	85	73	3·8	98	91	70	1·5
	Rural	100	93	11	0·0	96	90	25	3·7
Bladder	Copenhagen	99	94	69	0·8	98	91	74	1·8
	Rural	97	87	38	2·5	95	81	36	5·1
Hodgkin	Copenhagen	100	92	90	0·0	100	96	87	0·0
	Rural	98	93	61	2·4	98	93	70	2·0

cancer cases is diagnosed in hospitals in Copenhagen as in rural Denmark. However, slightly fewer cases in rural areas are histologically verified, and a much lower proportion of fatal cases in rural areas are autopsied. Asymptomatic tumours are thus less likely to be registered in rural areas than in Copenhagen, and tumour diagnosis is likely to be slightly less exact in rural Denmark. The basis for urban-rural comparisons is probably less favourable in many other countries.

Urban-rural differences in cancer morbidity

A systematic exploration of urban-rural differences in cancer morbidity is undertaken by a number of Cancer Registries. As an example, data from Denmark are shown in Table 3, giving the ratios

TABLE 3. Copenhagen-rural ratios of selected cancer sites in Denmark 1968-1972
(from Clemmesen, 1977)

Site	Males	Females
Lip	0·3	1·2
Mouth	2·3	1·3
Oesophagus	2·2	1·3
Stomach	1·0	0·9
Colon	1·8	1·2
Rectum	1·3	1·0
Liver	3·5	1·0
Pancreas	1·7	1·4
Larynx	2·5	2·8
Lung	3·0	2·2
Breast	—	1·3
Cervix uteri	—	1·5
Corpus uteri	—	1·2
Ovary	—	1·2
Prostate	1·3	—
Testis	1·2	—
Kidney	1·7	1·4
Bladder	2·1	2·0
Melanoma of Skin	1·2	1·3
Brain	0·8	1·2
Eye	1·0	1·0
Thyroid	1·3	0·9
Hodgkin's Disease	1·1	1·1
Leukaemia	1·0	1·0
All sites	1·6	1·3

of age-standardized rates between Copenhagen and rural areas (Clemmesen, 1977). Keeping the above-mentioned sources of error in mind, it appears that cancer occurs 60 per cent more frequently in males and 30 per cent more frequently in females in Copenhagen than in rural Denmark. Clear excess risks associated with living in Copenhagen are seen for the development of cancer of the oesophagus, colon, liver (males), pancreas, larynx, lung, cervix uteri, kidney and bladder. Other sites show no, or only slight, differences between Copenhagen and rural areas. With a few exceptions, similar trends are seen in other Scandinavian countries (Cancer Registry of Norway, 1973; Teppo et al., 1975).

An urban excess of cancer morbidity in general is also noted in England and Wales (Office of Population Census and Surveys, 1972), amounting to 30 per cent in males and 20 per cent in females. The figures for England and Wales indicate much less urban–rural variation for almost all sites compared with Scandinavia. Urban–rural differences in cancer mortality resembling the pattern described for Scandinavia were recently published for the United States by Hoover et al. (1975). Information on possible urban–rural variation in cancer in developing countries is not available.

Clues to Aetiology

Associations between cancer occurrence and a specific setting (affluent–poor society, urban-rural area) may indicate areas of aetiological importance by the identification of factors present in the environment in question. Affluence and urbanization may in general be seen as influencing humans in three ways by leading to: changes of personal habits (e.g., smoking, drinking, diet), changes in the occupational environment (e.g., industrialization) and changes in the general environment (e.g., pollution of air, water, food). Examples of the role of these changes in determining international as well as urban–rural variation in cancer occurrence will be given below.

Latency period

When relating differentials in cancer risk to environmental factors, both internationally and within countries, it must be borne in mind that both the measurements of cancer occurrence and the prevalence of the environmental factor under study usually represent isolated values of parameters which are often changing over time. The long latency period of some 20 to 40 years for cancer development must, if possible, be taken into account, and present-day cancer incidence or mortality thus reflects exposures starting, or occurring, around 1950.

Personal habits

A person's behaviour and habits are to a large extent ruled by his cultural environment and influenced by socially accepted norms. As far back as 1842, Rigoni Stern suggested that the higher rates of cancer among nuns in Verona should be sought in their particular way of life: "in the food they eat, and more particularly in the excessive use of fish and oil, or in the long and repeated fasts" and he asked about "the cause of the even more frequently found cancer of the breast. Is it perhaps the too-tight corsets, or the prolonged attitude of prayer with the forearms resting on the Prie-Dieu compressing the breasts?".

While research in the role of dietary factors in the aetiology of cancer has recently become more intensified, epidemiological cancer research, prompted by the rise in lung cancer frequency, has during recent decades been concentrated on the habit of smoking.

Tobacco

Tobacco smoking is associated with cancer of the mouth and upper respiratory-digestive tract, lung and bladder (Clemmesen, 1964, 1974; (Higginson and Jensen, 1977; UICC, 1976). It has been estimated that approximately 90 per cent of all cases of lung cancer can be attributed to smoking.

It was early demonstrated by Clemmesen and Nielsen (1955) that the international distribution of lung cancer is consistent with differences in smoking habits (Fig. 3). The urban excess of lung cancer (Table 3) has long been puzzling. It has often been related to the higher level of air pollution in cities as well as specific occupational exposures affecting a proportion of urban dwellers. The relative importance of smoking, air pollution and occupation in the aetiology of lung cancer has been discussed by the UICC (1976), who confirmed the overwhelming role of cigarette smoking, considered a slight proportion of cases — 'probably less than 5%' — to be attributable to occupation, and found little evidence of an aetiological role of present levels of air pollution.

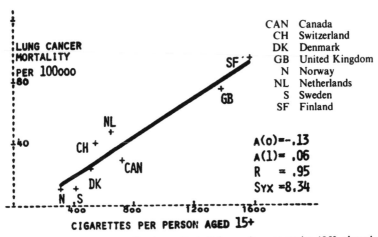

FIG. 3. Lung cancer mortality (age-adjusted) for various countries 1950 plotted against national annual cigarette consumption *per capita*, in 1930. (From Clemmesen, 1974.)

Table 4 shows that the urban–rural difference in smoking habits is an important variable, which must be taken into account when explaining urban–rural differences in lung cancer. There is a good correspondence between the ratios for lung cancer and proportion of the male population smoking cigarettes approximately 10 to 20 years earlier; no account has been taken of the fact that urban smokers on the average also smoke more cigarettes per day than rural smokers (Tobacco Research Council, 1972). It is interesting to note that urban excess of lung cancer has been only slight in Finland, where cigarette smoking was widespread both in urban and rural communities around the turn of the century (Pernu, 1960).

TABLE 4. Urban–rural ratios of lung cancer and cigarette consumption among males

	Denmark Copenhagen–rural	Finland urban–rural	England and Wales conurbations–rural
Lung cancer*	3·0	1·2	1·5
Cigarettes†	2·8	1·0	1·1

* Denmark incidence 1968–72 (Clemmesen, 1977); Finland incidence 1966–70 (Teppo *et al.*, 1975); England and Wales mortality 1970.
† Denmark 1953 (Morbiditetsundersøgelsen af 1950, 1960); Finland 1962 (Pedersen *et al.*, 1969); England and Wales 1952 (Tobacco Research Council, 1972).

The difference in air pollution between Copenhagen and rural Denmark is much less than between conurbations and rural areas in England and Wales, contrasting with the much higher urban–rural ratios for lung cancer in Denmark than in England (Table 4).

Alcohol

Tobacco smoking interacts with alcohol in the production of cancer of the mouth, pharynx, larynx and oesophagus in developed countries, as reviewed by Clemmesen (1964). Although oesophageal cancer occurs more often in urban than in rural areas in Northern Europe and North America (Table 3), this association with urbanization is not uniform and should not be taken to indicate an unidentified 'urban' factor of aetiological importance. In Northern France oesophageal cancer is thus predominantly a rural disease (Tuyns and Massé, 1975 a, b). Data from France and Denmark (Table 5) show that these opposite urban–rural differences are consistent with trends in alcohol consumption.

TABLE 5. Cancer of the oesophagus and alcohol consumption among males

Area	C. oesophagus rate per 100 000*	Daily alcohol consumption (g)†
Denmark		
Copenhagen	7·4	31
Rural areas	3·4	12
Ille-et-Vilaine, France		
Urban cantons	27·7	37
Rural cantons	42·8	48

* Denmark: age-standardized to 'European' population (Clemmesen, 1977).
  France: not age-standardized (estimated from Tuyns and Massé, 1975 b).
† Figures not comparable between Denmark (International Agency for Research on Cancer, 1978) and France (Tuyns *et al.*, 1975).

In other parts of the world, other habits are associated with these diseases. For example, the high incidence of cancer of the mouth and oesophagus in India (Fig. 1) is associated with the habit of betel-nut chewing. The high incidence of oesophageal cancer in Iran is unrelated to alcohol, and probably associated with some other, as yet, unidentified way of life (Joint Iran–International Agency for Research on Cancer, 1977).

Composition of diet

Dietary habits other than alcohol drinking also vary both internationally and within countries between town and countryside as well as between different social strata. High dietary fat intake (Aries *et al.*, 1969) and fibre deficiency in the diet (Burkitt, 1969) have been associated with cancer of the large bowel, one of the most frequent cancers in the developed part of the world. This dietary pattern is typical of Europe, North America and Australasia, and studies of Japanese migrants to the United States have shown that their risk increases with a shift from a low to a high incidence setting (Haenszel, 1961). The concentration of cocarcinogenic metabolites of bile acids is associated with the incidence of colon cancer (Hill *et al.*, 1971), and the level of bile acid is, in turn, believed to be determined by the intake of fat (Hill, 1975).

A more complex pattern involving both the faecal content of carcinogens or cocarcinogens and a protective effect of dietary fibre, has recently been suggested (International Agency for Research on Cancer, 1977).

Further investigations of the role of diet in cancer development are indicated, examining both the possible turnover-initiating or promoting effects of ingested substances, e.g., fat/meat and colon cancer, nitrate and stomach cancer (*Lancet*, 1977), and the 'risk modifying' effect of dietary substances, e.g., dietary fibre and colon cancer, vitamin A and lung cancer (Bjelke, 1975).

Occupational environment

Occupational exposure to a number of substances is associated with an increased risk of developing cancer of the gastro-intestinal tract, liver, nasal cavities, larynx, lung, bladder, skin, bone and haematopoietic system, as listed in Table 6. These hazards are, in turn, associated with urbanization through industrialization, and they thereby contribute to the cancer patterns observed in the developed parts of the world, as well as to the urban–rural differences. Present estimates of the proportion of all cancers attributable to occupational hazards vary from less than 5 per cent up to 'less than' 15 per cent (Higginson and Muir, 1976; Cole, 1977). Although the direct contribution to the total amount of cancer in society may thus be limited, the identification of industrially related cancers is important as a basis for undertaking preventive measures (e.g.,

TABLE 6.   Agents involving occupational exposure and an increased risk of cancer

Site	Agent
Gastro-intestinal tract	Asbestos
Liver	Vinyl chloride
Nasal cavity	Isopropyl oils, nickel,
Sinuses	Wood and leather dusts
Larynx	Isopropyl oils, mustard gas
Lung	Arsenic, asbestos, bis(chloromethyl)ether, chromium, haematite mining, mustard gas, nickel, soot, tars, oils ionizing radiation
Pleura, peritoneum	Asbestos
Bladder	4-aminobiphenyl, benzidine, 2-naphthylamine
Skin	Arsenic, ionizing radiation, soot, tars, oils
Bone	Ionizing radiation
Haematopoietic system	Benzene, ionizing radiation

change of process, introduction of hygienic standards) of importance for the workers involved. Furthermore, low-level exposure of larger population groups may occur, increasing the public health problem even if the relative risk is lower than in industry.

Interaction with personal habits, e.g. cigarette smoking and asbestos in lung cancer (Saracci, 1977), does occur, but such interaction is unknown for the majority of substances listed (Table 6).

General environment

Increasing affluence and industrialization modify the general environment to which humans are exposed. Discharge of chemicals pollutes the air, and industrialized food production has led to the use of food additives and food preservatives. General hygienic standards relating to food and water in affluent societies have undoubtedly played a major role in diminishing many acute conditions, but the chemical pollution of our environment as a possible cause of chronic illness has raised concern.

General air pollution has been incriminated in the production of lung cancer, but attempts to establish such a relationship have not been very satisfactory. The role of air pollution has been difficult to assess, owing to the overwhelming role of cigarette smoking. The importance of differences in cigarette consumption in the urban–rural ratios for lung cancer has been mentioned above (Table 4). Exposure to coal tar in the general environment might be expected to increase the risk of lung cancer, yet the risk of lung cancer in gas workers has been found to be only about 1·5 times higher than in the general population in spite of a more than 100-fold excess in benz(a)pyrene levels in the air breathed by these workers compared with the level to which the total urban population is exposed (Waller, 1972).

City air contains low concentrations of known carcinogens and exposure to such concentrations apparently has no effect in non-smokers. There is, thus, at present no indication that general air pollution *per se* causes lung cancer; the possibility that it interacts with cigarette smoking to increase the risk in smokers needs further investigation, however. Data from a prospective investigation in Sweden are suggestive of this latter possibility (Cederlöf *et al.*, 1975; Friberg and Cederlöf, 1978) but more observations are needed before any conclusions can be drawn.

Conclusions

Cancer occurs frequently in both the developed and undeveloped parts of the world, but constitutes at present a larger public health problem in the former. Cancers at specific sites show in general larger international variation than all cancers taken together, and a number of aetiological factors have been identified in both rich and poor societies.

Cancer occurs on average slightly more frequently in affluent than in poor societies and in urban rather than rural areas of the former. It may be concluded that the frequency of numerically important cancer sites in developed countries and in urban areas is to a large extent determined by personal habits. Occupational exposure *per se* is probably less important, and the role of low-dose exposure to carcinogens in the general environment is largely undetermined, but available data suggest that such exposures are relatively unimportant in cancer development. Possible interactions between personal habits, occupational exposure and the general environment in the development of cancer needs further study.

References

ARIES, V., CROWTHER, J. S., DRASAR, B. S., HILL, M. J. and WILLIAMS, R. E. O. (1969) Bacteria and the aetiology of cancer of the large bowel. *Gut*, 10, 334–335.

BJELKE, E. (1975) Dietary vitamin A and human lung cancer. *International Journal of Cancer*, 15, 561–565.

BURKITT, D. P. (1969) Related disease—related cause? *Lancet*, ii, 1229–1231.

CANCER REGISTRY OF NORWAY (1973) *Cancer Registration in Norway. The Incidence of Cancer in Norway, 1969–1971*. Oslo: Norwegian Cancer Society.

CEDERLÖF, R., FRIBERG, L., HRUBEC, Z. and LORICH, U. (1975) *The Relationship of Smoking and some Social Covariables to Mortality and Cancer Morbidity*. Parts I and II. Stockholm: Department of Environmental Hygiene, Karolinska Institute.

CLEMMESEN, J. (1964) Statistical studies in the aetiology of malignant neoplasms, Vol. I. *Acta pathologica et microbiologica scandinavica*, Suppl., 174.

CLEMMESEN, J. (1974) Statistical studies in the aetiology of malignant neoplasms, Vol. IV. *Acta pathologica et microbiologica scandinavica*, Suppl., 247.

CLEMMESEN, J. (1977) Statistical studies in the aetiology of malignant neoplasms, Vol. V. *Acta pathologica et microbiologica scandinavica*, Suppl., 261.

CLEMMESEN, J. and NIELSEN, A. (1955) The geographical and racial distribution of cancer of the lung. *Schweizerische Zeitschrift für Pathologie und Bakteriologie*, 18, 803–819.

COLE, P. (1977) Cancer and occupation: Status and needs of epidemiologic research. *Cancer*, 39, 1788–1791.

DAY, N. E. (1976) A new measure of age-standardized incidence, the cumulative rate. In *Cancer Incidence in Five Continents*, Vol. III, eds. WATERHOUSE, J. A. H., MUIR, C. S., CORREA, P. and POWELL, J. Lyons: IARC Scientific Publication No. 15, International Agency for Research on Cancer.

DOLL, R. (1969) The geographical distribution of cancer. *British Journal of Cancer*, 23, 1–8.

DOLL, R. (1976) Comparisons between registries. Age-standardized rates. *Cancer Incidence in Five Continents*, Vol. III, eds. WATERHOUSE, J. A. H., MUIR, C. S., CORREA, P. and POWELL, J. Lyons: IARC Scientific Publication No. 15, International Agency for Research on Cancer.

DOLL, R. and COOK, P. (1967) Summarising indices for comparison of cancer incidence data. *International Journal of Cancer*, 2, 269–279.

FREDERICI, N., PRIGUANO, A. S., PASQUALI, P., CARIANI, G. and NATALE, M. (1976) Urban–rural differences in mortality, 1950–1970. *World Health Statistics Report*, 29, 249–378.

FRIBERG, L. and CEDERLÖF, R. (1978) Late effects of air pollution with special reference to lung cancer. *Environmental Health Perspectives*, 22, 45—66.

HAENSZEL, W. (1961) Cancer mortality among the foreign-born in the United States. *Journal of the National Cancer Institute*, 26, 37–132.

HIGGINSON, J. and JENSEN, O. M. (1977) Epidemiological review of lung cancer in man. In *Air Pollution and Cancer in Man*, eds. MÖHR, U., SCHMÄHL, D. and TOMATIS, L. Lyons: IARC Scientific Publication No. 16, International Agency for Research on Cancer.

HIGGINSON, J. and MUIR, C. S. (1976) The role of epidemiology in elucidating the importance of environmental factors in human cancer. *Cancer Detection and Prevention*, 1, 79–105.

HILL, M. J. (1975) Etiology of colon cancer. *CRC Critical Review of Toxicology*, 4, 31–82.

HILL, M. J., CROWTHER, J. S., DRASAR, B. S., HAWKSWORTH, G., ARIES, V. C. and WILLIAMS, R. E. O. (1971) Bacteria and aetiology of cancer of the large bowel. *Lancet*, i, 95–99.

HOOVER, R., MASON, T. J., MCKAY, F. W. and FRAUMENI, J. F. (1975) Geographic patterns of cancer mortality in the United States. In *Persons at High Risk of Cancer*, ed. FRAUMENI, J. F. New York: Academic Press.

INTERNATIONAL AGENCY OF RESEARCH ON CANCER, Intestinal Microecology Group (1977) Dietary fibre, transit time, faecal bacteria, steroids and colon cancer in two Scandinavian populations. *Lancet*, ii, 207–211.

INTERNATIONAL AGENCY FOR RESEARCH ON CANCER, Intestinal Microecology Group (1978) Personal communication.

JENSEN, O. M., MOSBECH, J., SALASPURO, M. and IHAMÄKI, T. (1974) A comparative study of the diagnostic basis for cancer of the colon and cancer of the rectum in Denmark and Finland. *International Journal of Epidemiology*, 3, 183–186.

JOINT IRAN–INTERNATIONAL AGENCY FOR RESEARCH ON CANCER STUDY GROUP (1977) Esophageal cancer studies in the Caspian Littoral of Iran: Results of population studies. A prodrome. *Journal of the National Cancer Institute*, 59, 1127–1138.

Lancet (1977) Nitrate and human cancer. *Lancet*, ii, 281–282.

MORBIDITETSUNDERSØGELSEN AF 1950 (1960) *Sygdomsundersøgelsen i Danmark 1951–1954*. Copenhagen: Munksgaard.

OFFICE OF POPULATION CENSUSES AND SURVEYS (1972) *The Registrar General's Statistical Review of England and Wales for the Two Years 1966–1967. Supplement on Cancer*. London: H.M.S.O.

PEDERSEN, E., MAGNUS, K., MORK, T., HOUGEN, A., BJELKE, E., HAKAMA, M. and SAXÉN, E. (1969) Lung cancer in Finland and Norway: an epidemiological study. *Acta pathologica et microbiologica scandinavica*, Suppl., 199.

PERNU, J. (1960) An epidemiological study on cancer of the digestive tract and respiratory system: a study based on 7078 cases. *Annales Medicinae Internae Fenniae*, Suppl. 33, 1–117.

SARACCI, R. (1977) Asbestos and lung cancer. An analysis of the epidemiological evidence on the asbestos–smoking interaction. *International Journal of Cancer*, 20, 323–331.

SEGI, M. and KURIHARA, M (1960–72) Cancer mortality for selected sites in 24 countries. *Japanese Cancer Society*, 1–6.

STERN, R. (1842) Fatti statistici relativi alle malattie cancerose. *Giornale per servire ai progresi della patologia e della terapeutica. Serie II*, 2, 507–517.

TEPPO, L., HAKAMA, M., HAKULINEN, T., LEHTONEN, M. and SAXÉN, E. (1975) Cancer in Finland 1953–1970. Incidence, mortality, prevalence. *Acta pathologica et microbiologica scandinavica*, Suppl., 252.

TOBACCO RESEARCH COUNCIL (1972) *Statistics of Smoking in the United Kingdom*. Research paper I, 6th edn. London: Tobacco Research Council.

TUYNS, A. J. and MASSÉ, G. (1975 a) Cancer of the oesophagus in Brittany: an incidence study in Ille-et-Vilaine. *International Journal of Epidemiology*, 4, 55–59.

TUYNS, A. J. and MASSÉ, G. (1975 b) Le cancer de l'oesophage en Ille-et-Vilaine. Etude de l'incidence de la maladie, des ses aspects cliniques et histologiques et de sa distribution géographique. *Ouest Médicale*, 28, 1757–1770.

TUYNS, A. J., PEQUIGNOT, G., JENSEN, O. M. and POMEAU, Y. (1975) La consommation individuelle de boissons alcoolisées et de tabac dans un échantillon de la population en Ille-et-Vilaine. *Révue de l'alcool*, 21, 1–46.

TUYNS, A. J. and RAVISSE, P. (1970) Cancer in Brazzaville, the Congo. *Journal of the National Cancer Institute*, 4, 1121–1127.

UICC (1976) Lung cancer. *UICC Technical Report Series*, Vol. 25. Geneva: Union Internationale Contre le Cancer.

WALLER, R. E. (1972) The combined effects of smoking and occupational or urban factors in relation to lung cancer. *Annals of Occupational Hygiene*, 15, 67–71.

WATERHOUSE, J. A. H., MUIR, C. S., CORREA, P. and POWELL, J. (eds.) (1976) *Cancer Incidence in Five Continents*, Vol. III. Lyons: IARC Scientific Publication No. 15, International Agency for Research on Cancer.

WORLD HEALTH ORGANIZATION (1967) *International Statistical Classification of Diseases, Injuries and Causes of Death*, 8th Revision. Geneva: World Health Organization.

WORLD HEALTH ORGANIZATION (1978) *World Health Statistics. Vital Statistics and Causes of Death*, Vol. I. Geneva: World Health Organization.

AFFLUENCE, URBANIZATION AND CORONARY HEART DISEASE

M. G. MARMOT

Department of Medical Statistics and Epidemiology,
London School of Hygiene and Tropical Medicine

'CONCLUSIONS' about the nature of coronary heart disease (CHD) abound. It is commonly stated, and presumably believed, that: (1) CHD is a disease of affluence; (2) CHD is associated with a modern, urban way of life; (3) in particular, the modern epidemic of CHD is associated with a diet rich in saturated fat, with smoking and with a sedentary life-style.

This is a graphic picture of CHD. It conjures up notions of our paying the price for living in large stressful non-human cities, over-indulging in food and tobacco, and leading lazy sedentary lives. Neat and credible as is this concept of the causes of CHD, it is too simple a picture. Each of the above 'conclusions' bears further examination, in both developed and developing countries. It will be seen that they hold only under certain circumstances.

CHD as a Disease of Affluence

Every 10 years in England and Wales the Registrar-General reports mortality in different social classes — the classification into classes is based on occupation. Table 1, taken from the 1971 Decennial Supplement of Occupational Mortality (Office of Population Censuses and Surveys, 1978) shows the standardized mortality ratio for CHD in the standard five classes. It is clear that classes I and II, the most affluent, have the lowest mortality from

127

TABLE 1.   Ischaemic heart disease mortality (SMR) by social class, men. England and
Wales 1970–1972.*

Social class	Standardized mortality ratio
I	88
II	91
III non-manual	114
III manual	107
IV	108
V	111

* Occupational Mortality, Office of Population Censuses and Surveys (1978).

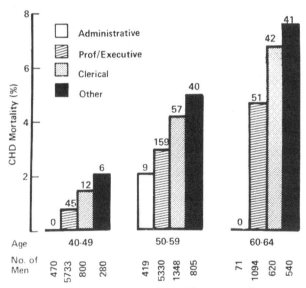

FIG. 1.   Coronary heart disease mortality in $7\frac{1}{2}$ years by civil service grade and age
(Marmot et al., 1978 b).

CHD. Further support for this inverse association between social
class and CHD mortality comes from a longitudinal study of civil
servants working in Whitehall, in London. Men were classified
according to their grade of employment and followed for $7\frac{1}{2}$ years
(Fig. 1). The CHD death rate among men in the lowest grade was
nearly four times that among men in the highest (administrative)
grade (Marmot et al., 1978 b).

We were intrigued by this apparent conflict between the popular prejudice of CHD as the rich man's disease and the data, and we recently examined the association between CHD mortality and social class in England and Wales at different points in time (Marmot *et al.*, 1978 a). Allowing for changes in diagnostic fashion, it appears that deaths from CHD *were* more common in upper-class men until 1951. By 1961 the rate for upper-class men had begun to level off, but the rates for working class men had continued to rise and had overtaken the rates in classes I and II. Working-class women have never "had it so very good". Their death rates from heart disease were higher than those of women in class I and II throughout the period of study (1931–1971).

What we are seeing in England and Wales is a changing pattern. CHD may have been predominantly a disease of affluence during the period when CHD mortality was rapidly increasing. It is no longer either rapidly increasing or a disease of the most affluent.

A similar picture emerges if we examine ethnic differences in the USA. Clinical teaching had it that CHD was less common among blacks than among whites. Fig. 2 shows CHD mortality for blacks and whites aged 50 to 54 in the USA for 1962 (Stamler, 1967). For men, the CHD death rates are very similar. In women, blacks have a

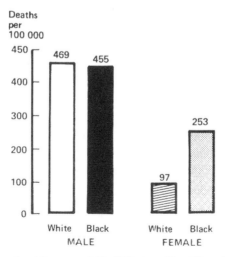

FIG. 2.   Coronary heart disease mortality USA at age 50 to 54 by colour and sex, 1962 (Stamler, 1967).

higher CHD mortality than whites. Once again, these data appear to conflict with popular prejudice. It is possible that this is analogous to the CHD distribution among the social classes in Britain. At an earlier stage of America's social and economic history, before there was a large migration of blacks from the rural south into the cities of the north. CHD may have been relatively more common among whites. Support for this is provided by a longitudinal study of CHD incidence from Evans County in Georgia, USA (Cassel, 1971). In this largely rural population, the blacks still work as farm labourers and sharecroppers under poor conditions. The CHD incidence over 7 years of follow-up is shown in Fig. 3. For both males and females the incidence rate is higher among whites.

To the extent that the CHD differences between blacks and whites are related to socio-economic factors, this is consistent with the picture in Britain. When the whole population has gone beyond a certain level of economic development, CHD is no longer a disease limited to the more affluent members of society.

If this were true, one might expect that in poorer countries CHD would be still a disease of the more affluent. There is a shortage of population studies of vascular disease from developing countries, but

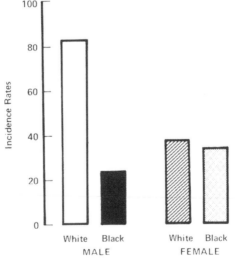

FIG. 3. CHD incidence/1000 in 7 years (age-adjusted) by colour and sex — Evans County, USA (Cassel 1971).

such data as we have support this. A study in Northern India found CHD to be more common among wealthier people (Sarvotham and Berry, 1968). In South Africa, CHD is more common among whites than among blacks, i.e., the coronary disease pattern is more like rural Georgia than industrial USA (Shaper, 1973).

The first 'conclusion' must, therefore, be modified. In general, CHD is more common in affluent countries than in poor countries, although there are some exceptions. Within less affluent countries it is the wealthier members of society who appear to be at highest risk; within wealthy countries CHD is more common among the poorer members of society.

CHD as a Disease of a Modern Urban Life

In examining this proposition, one might ask if CHD is more frequent in urban areas than rural areas. I propose to look at this question in countries at three different stages of development: (1) Britain, representing the urbanized industrialized world; (2) countries at an intermediate stage such as Yugoslavia and Puerto Rico; and (3) in developing countries. Table 2 shows the Standardized Mortality Ratios for ischaemic heart disease in England and Wales (1969–1973) according to degree of urbanization. These unpublished data were kindly made available by Dr. A. Adelstein of the Office of Population Censuses and Surveys. The CHD mortality is slightly lower in rural areas of the country than in towns and cities. In urban areas there is no association between size of city and CHD mortality. One is very tempted to post H.M. Government Health Department's warnings: "Cities can seriously damage your health", opposite the cigarette

TABLE 2. Ischaemic heart disease mortality.* England and Wales 1969–1973.

	Standard mortality ratio	
	Males	Females
Conurbations	102	99
Urban ≥ 100 000	104	104
Urban 50 000–99 999	100	99
Urban < 50 000	103	102
Rural	92	97

* Unpublished data of Dr. Adelstein, Office of Population Censuses and Surveys.

advertisements. In Britain, the data for CHD distribution scarcely provide the evidence for the hazards of urban life.

If we move to countries lower down the scale of urbanization and development, the picture is somewhat different. In Yugoslavia, a longitudinal study has shown that CHD incidence is nearly twice as high among urban residents as among rural residents (Kozarevic et al., 1976). Similar data have come from Puerto Rico (Garcia-Palmieri et al., 1978). We might consider these countries to be at an intermediate stage of development: not as urbanized and 'developed' as Northern Europe and North America, but more so than the developing countries of Asia and Africa.

In the developing world there are few data one can point to on urban–rural differences in CHD occurrence. However, several studies have been performed on the distribution of blood pressure and other coronary risk factors. In interpreting these data a caution is in order. Blood pressure is a major risk factor for coronary heart disease. In countries where the overall level of CHD risk is low, however, high blood pressure does not carry the same absolute risk of CHD as it does in high risk countries. Nevertheless, development of high blood pressure is likely to be one step further towards the development of CHD.

It has now commonly been reported that there are communities whose members have low average levels of blood pressure, and in whom the level of blood pressure does not rise with age. These communities are, almost without exception, rural, traditional in their culture and have little contact with the outside world (Henry and Cassel, 1969). The fact that such communities are to be found in parts of Africa is of great interest, as blacks in the USA have very high average levels of blood pressure and show a steep rise with age. To show the contrast, Vaughan and Miall (1978) compared the data from several studies in Africa with a study of people in Jamaica of African ancestry. Data on blood pressure and age from these comparisons are presented in Fig. 4. It should be noted that there is a danger in comparing blood pressures from different studies because of variability in the methods of measurement. In the present case, this variability should have been minimal because the same investigator, Dr. Miall, supervised the blood pressure measurements in all three studies. The studies in The Gambia and Tanzania were carried out in isolated rural areas. The Jamaican study took place in a farming area

SYSTOLIC BLOOD PRESSURE – AFRICANS (MALES)

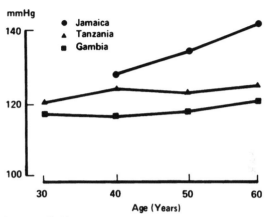

FIG. 4.   Mean systolic blood pressure by age in three populations of men (Vaughan and Miall, 1978).

close to the capital city of Kingston, with which there was regular communication. Blood pressures in The Gambia and Tanzania are low and there is little rise with age. By contrast, the Jamaicans had higher pressures and a clear rise of blood pressure with age. A similar picture is seen for females. The average blood pressures for blacks in the USA are likely to be higher than the Jamaican figures.

When the blood pressures of rural, unacculturated groups have been compared with more urbanized groups in developing countries in Asia and the Pacific, there have been similar findings: higher blood pressure in the more urbanized. When making these comparisons one must ask if the groups are comparable in respects other than their degree of urbanization, e.g., might the groups being compared be genetically different? One approach to this question is provided by the study of migrants. This may be illustrated by the Tokelau Island Migrant Study conducted by Prior and his colleagues (Prior, et al., 1974). The Tokelau islanders are Polynesians living on Pacific atolls just south of the equator. Because of population pressure on the atolls there has been a continued migration of the islanders to New Zealand. Surveys of the Tokelauans have been carried out both on the islands and in New Zealand where they live mainly in the cities. Representative results for systolic blood pressure are shown in Fig. 5.

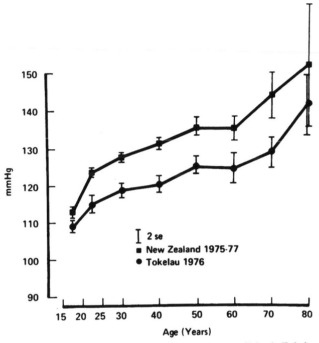

FIG. 5.   Mean systolic blood pressure by age for Tokelau men living in Tokelau and in New Zealand (I.A.M. Prior *et al.*, unpublished data).

Both the migrants in New Zealand and the Tokelauans on the islands show a rise of blood pressure with age. The blood pressures of the migrants are significantly higher, 10 mm Hg or more, than the blood pressures of the islanders.

These results are certainly consistent with an urban–rural difference in vascular disease in developing countries. They are, however, subject to the criticism levelled at all migrant studies: that migrants may be different from non-migrants in ways other than having chosen to migrate. It must be asked if the migrants are a special population, liable to hypertension. Prior and his colleagues have answered this question in a unique way by conducting a prospective study of the Tokelauans. They measured pressures of the potential migrants while still resident on the islands and followed them in New Zealand. These were compared with Tokelauans who remained resident on the islands, i.e. non-migrants. The blood

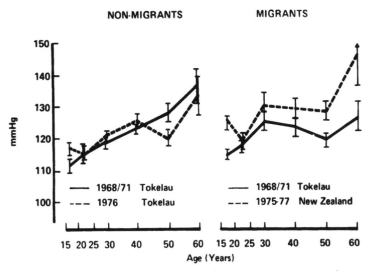

NON-MIGRANTS   **MIGRANTS**

FIG. 6. Mean systolic blood pressure by age for Tokelauan men comparing non-migrants and men who subsequently migrated to New Zealand (Prior *et al.*, unpublished data).

pressures of the non-migrants and migrants are shown in Fig. 6 (I.A.M. Prior, unpublished data). Both groups had blood pressure readings taken between 1968 and 1971 on the islands. The follow-up readings were taken an average of 6 years later, on the islands for the non-migrants, and in New Zealand for the migrants. While on the islands, the non-migrants and the pre-migrants had similar levels of blood pressure. Six years later, the blood pressures of the migrants had risen, to a greater extent than the blood pressures of the non-migrants. Similar changes have been found with plasma lipids.

Data on urban–rural differences have recently been published in the People's Republic of China (Cardiovascular Institute, 1978). One might wonder if the process of urbanization in China is different from other developing countries. It may be, but as seen in Table 3, the effect of urbanization on blood pressure appears to be similar. The data were reported as 'per cent hypertensive'. The more urban the population, the greater the proportion found on survey to be hypertensive.

If we put together the data on social class and urban–rural differences in CHD and blood pressure, we may start to build up a

Table 3. Prevalence rate (%) of hypertension in three Chinese communities.* Males and females combined.

	Age	
	40–49	50–59
Rural — Hopei	5·5%	9·1%
Peking suburb	10·2%	15·5%
Peking urban	18·1%	33·1%

*Cardiovascular Institute (1978).

picture. In developing countries it is the more wealthy urbanized groups who are at the highest risk of CHD. In the industrialized wealthy countries, if this pattern used to exist, it does no longer. The urban–rural differences in CHD are small and it is the poorer members of society who have the most vascular disease. As shown in the previous section, there is evidence that this is a new pattern in the affluent countries. It appears that the most recent groups to become urbanized and achieve a threshold level of economic development have the highest risk of CHD. Those newly exposed to the urban way of life are perhaps less able to adapt to the biological and social challenge.

Challenge of urbanization

There is some evidence to support this speculation, from countries at various levels of development. In South Africa it has been shown that Zulus living in urban areas have higher blood pressures than rural residents (Scotch, 1960). Among the urban residents, recent arrivals to the city had higher blood pressures than long-term residents (Scotch, 1963).

Similar results for CHD incidence have been reported from the study in Puerto Rico, that was taken to illustrate a country at an intermediate stage of development (García-Palmieri et al., 1978). In that study, urban residents had a greater CHD incidence rate than rural residents. Fig. 7 shows the CHD incidence rates with the subjects classified according to the length of time they had lived in the urban area under study. The numbers in some of these subgroups were fairly small, and the confidence intervals around the rates are large. There is the suggestion that the more recent arrivals to the city had a higher CHD incidence than the long-term residents.

PUERTO RICO

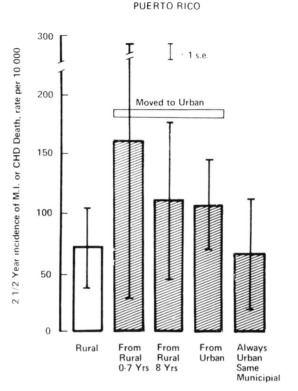

Fig. 7.   CHD incidence among urban and rural residents by migration status—
Puerto Rico (Garcia-Palmieri *et al.*, 1978).

In the USA, Tyroler and Cassel (1964) tackled this problem in a different way. They were interested in CHD mortality, not in the case when people came to the city, but in the case where the city came to the people. To do this, in the predominantly rural state of North Carolina, they studied rural residents who lived in counties that were becoming progressively more urbanized as the cities continued to grow (Fig. 8). The 100 counties in North Carolina were classified on a four-point scale from 'least urban' (1), to 'most urban' (4) depending on the size of the largest city. Data are shown for the western half of the state, the part with the most rapid increase in industrialization between the two time periods shown. In the earlier time period, the more urbanized the area, the higher was the CHD mortality among

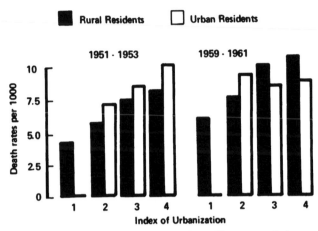

FIG. 8. CHD death rates, white males 55 to 64 by residence status (urban–rural) and index of urbanization (1 is least and 4 is most urbanized) (Tyroler and Cassel, 1964).

both urban and rural residents of the area. In the later period, for rural residents there was still an association between degree of urbanization of the county and CHD mortality. This was no longer true for urban residents. Furthermore, the urban–rural difference in CHD—higher in urban—that was apparent in the earlier period was no longer in evidence in 1959–1961. Thus these data are consistent with two observations: (1) rural residents living in areas that have become largely urbanized have higher CHD rates than rural residents less affected by urbanization; (2) as urbanization has increased, rural residents have lost their apparent protection from CHD when compared with urban residents. It is those newly exposed to urbanization who appear to be at highest risk.

Searching for Causes: CHD, Fatty Diet, Smoking and Sedentary Life-style

I have been developing the thesis that it is only in situations of newly emerging urbanization or economic development that urbanization and affluence increase the risk of CHD. One must consider, however, what comprises the challenges posed by urbanization. Is it the exposure to a different diet? To smoking? To a sedentary life-style?

It is not the present intention to review exhaustively the epidemiology of CHD. Suffice to say that there is a large body of evidence linking a fatty diet, smoking and lack of physical activity to an increased risk of CHD. This is important and provides the basis for current efforts to prevent CHD. It is clear, however, that these factors explain only some part of the occurrence of CHD. Our understanding is far from complete. For example, in the study of social class and CHD in British Civil Servants, shown in Fig. 1, less than half of the CHD difference between the classes could be attributed to differences in smoking, blood pressure, plasma cholesterol or obesity (Marmot *et al.*, 1978 b).

The epidemiological study of CHD cross-culturally, in countries at varying levels of development, helps to sharpen the focus — to point to unexplained differences and to point to possible aetiological factors. I should like to illustrate this with examples from the study of diet and CHD.

There are probably no well-documented exceptions to the rule that countries with a high rate of CHD have a national diet that is rich in saturated fat. Despite the fact that these countries show other characteristics in common, it is difficult to avoid the possibility that the high CHD rate is related to the high level of consumption of saturated fat. The reverse is not necessarily true: populations with a high level of consumption of saturated fat may not have a high rate of

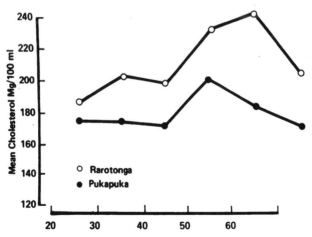

FIG. 9.   Mean serum cholesterol in two groups of Cook Islanders. Raratonga — most urbanized, and Pukapuka — less urbanized (Prior *et al.*, 1966).

CHD. Dramatic examples of this come from the studies of Polynesian islanders. In a companion study to the Tokelau Island Migrant Study, Prior *et al.* (1966) studied two groups of Polynesians living in the Cook Islands (Fig. 9). Rarotonga is the administrative capital of the Cook Islands and the group living there were relatively urbanized. Pukapuka is a remote coral atoll; its residents are much more cut off from the outside world. Fig. 9 shows the mean serum cholesterol levels of the two groups. If urbanization is related to risk of CHD, the plasma cholesterol levels are in the predicted direction—higher in the more urbanized Rarotongans. The interesting point comes with the examination of the dietary patterns of the two groups. The group with the low plasma cholesterol levels, the Pukapukans, consumed a diet that relies heavily on coconuts. Consequently, the Pukapukans have a much higher saturated fat consumption than the more urbanized Rarotongans, who consume more refined carbohydrates. Similarly, the coconut-eating Tokelauans decrease their saturated fat consumption when they migrate to New Zealand, but their serum lipid levels show a rise.

Burkitt and others have argued that we are looking at the wrong component of the diet: the reasons for the increasing rate of CHD and other diseases consequent upon urbanization is not too much fat

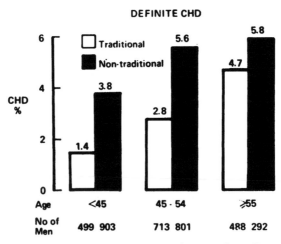

Fig. 10.   Culture of upbringing and prevalence of coronary heart disease in Japanese–Americans (Marmot and Syme, 1976).

consumed, but too little dietary fibre. It is an attractive hypothesis with as yet only scanty data to support or refute it. It would be wrong to set up a competition of fibre versus fat. It is quite possible that both types of dietary change may play a role in the development of CHD. Certainly neither factor alone accounts for many of the urban–rural, rich–poor differences in CHD to which reference has been made above.

These epidemiological studies of populations undergoing change may be used to study changes other than dietary ones. As an illustration I should like to refer briefly to one of our studies of Japanese migrants to the USA. Despite being highly urbanized and highly industrialized, Japan continues to have a low rate of CHD. When Japanese migrate to the USA their risk of CHD is intermediate between the high level of the Americans and the low level of Japanese in Japan. One obvious possible reason for the change in CHD rate is change in dietary fat consumption. This change in fat did not provide a complete explanation for the change in CHD occurrence (Marmot et al., 1975). We were interested to test the hypothesis that Japanese culture might in some way protect against the stress that increases CHD risk. To test this we concentrated our attention on the Japanese of California. Using a variety of techniques we classified them according to the degree to which they retained their traditional Japanese culture. The results of one such analysis are shown in Fig. 10, for an index that we labelled culture of upbringing. Californian Japanese who had been brought up in a more traditionally Japanese way had a lower CHD prevalence than men who were brought up in a less traditional pattern. This difference could not be explained by differences in dietary pattern, smoking, blood pressure or plasma cholesterol levels (Marmot and Syme, 1976). We had some evidence that this apparently protective effect was related to the level of support obtained from other members of the ethnic group.

Conclusions

One should be wary of generalizations about cities, and about affluent life-style. What is true in developing countries is not necessarily true in affluent countries. We need to know not only what it is about modern, affluent, urban life that may be related to CHD, but for how long people have experienced it. What emerges is the notion of a threshold of economic development below which CHD remains uncommon. Within a country, the groups who have reached the threshold more recently are at higher risk of CHD.

In the affluent countries, there appears to have been a process of adaptation. In the USA the rate of CHD mortality has now been declining for several years. In England and Wales it is only people in classes IV and V who continue to show an increase in CHD. For British doctors, and possibly for other men in classes I and II, the CHD rate has been declining (Doll and Peto, 1976). Whether this is a process of adaptation and exactly what it involves are not clear. It may be as comparatively simple as learning about hazards of certain habits, and voluntarily stopping smoking, putting on running shoes on a frosty morning, and cutting down on consumption of saturated fat and refined carbohydrates. It may be more subtle and related to learning to cope with the stresses of urban life. Whatever combination of these and other factors is crucial, it appears that we have two choices: either sit back and wait for the wave of the CHD epidemic to eventually pass through the population regardless of our efforts; or use the lessons to be learnt from the experience of the more affluent to attempt to prevent the 'luxury' of CHD being the inevitable consequence of economic development.

References

CARDIOVASCULAR INSTITUTE, Chinese Academy of Medical Sciences (1978) Community control of hypertension, stroke and coronary heart disease in a People's commune. *Chinese Medical Journal*, 4, 257–260.

CASSEL, J. C. (1971) Summary of major findings of the Evans County cardiovascular studies. *Archives of Internal Medicine*, 128, 887–889.

DOLL, R. and PETO, R. (1976) Mortality in relation to Smoking: 20 years' observations on male British doctors. *British Medical Journal*, 2, 1525–1536.

GARCIA-PALMIERI, M. R., COSTAS, R., JR., CRUZ-VIDAL, M., CORTÉS-ALICEA, M., PATTERNE, D., ROJAS-FRANCO, L., SORLIE, P. D. and KANNEL, W. B. (1978) Urban–rural differences in coronary heart disease in a low incidence area: the Puerto Rico heart disease in a low incidence area: the Puerto Rico heart study. *American Journal of Epidemiology*, 107, 206–215.

HENRY, J. P. and CASSEL, J. C. (1969) Psychosocial factors in essential hypertension. *American Journal of Epidemiology*, 90, 171–200.

KOZAREVIC, D., PIRC, B., RACIA, Z., DAWBER, T. R., GORDON, T. and ZUKEL, W. J. (1976) The Yugoslavia cardiovascular disease study II. Factors in the incidence of coronary heart disease. *American Journal of Epidemiology*, 104, 133–140.

MARMOT, M. G., ADELSTEIN, A., ROBINSON, N. and ROSE, G. (1978 a) Changing social class distribution of heart disease. *British Medical Journal*, 2, 1109–1112.

MARMOT, M. G., ROSE, G., SHIPLEY, M. and HAMILTON, P. J. S. (1978 b) Employment grade and coronary heart disease in British civil servants. *Journal of Epidemiology and Community Health*, 32 (in the press).

MARMOT, M. G. and SYME, S. L. (1976) Acculturation and coronary heart disease in Japanese-Americans. *American Journal of Epidemiology*, **104**, 225–247.

MARMOT, M. G., SYME, S. L., KAGAN, A., KATO, H., COHEN, J. B. and BELSKY, J. (1975) Epidemiologic studies of coronary heart disease and stroke in Japanese men living in Japan, Hawaii and California: Prevalence of coronary and hypertensive heart disease and associated risk factors. *American Journal of Epidemiology*, **102**, 514–525.

OFFICE OF POPULATION CENSUSES AND SURVEYS (1978) *Occupational Mortality*. The Registrar-General's decennial supplement for England and Wales (1970–1972) Series DS No. 1. London: HMSO.

PRIOR, I. A. M., HARVEY, H. P. B., NEAVE, M. I. and DAVIDSON, F. (1966) The health of two groups of Cook Island Maoris. New Zealand Department of Health Special Report Series No. 26, Wellington.

PRIOR, I. A. M., STANHOPE, J. M., EVANS, J. G. and SALMOND, C. E. (1974) The Tokelau Island Migrant Study. *International Journal of Epidemiology*, **3**, 225–232.

SARVOTHAM, S. G. and BERRY, J. N. (1968) Prevalence of coronary heart disease in an urban population in northern India. *Circulation*, **37**, 939–953.

SCOTCH, N. (1960) A preliminary report on the relation of sociocultural factors to hypertension among the Zulu. *Annals of the New York Academy of Science*, **84**, 1000–1009.

SCOTCH, N. (1963) Sociocultural factors in the epidemiology of Zulu hypertension. *American Journal of Public Health*, **53**, 1205–1213.

SHAPER, A. G. (1973) Coronary heart disease. In *Cardiovascular Disease in the Tropics*, eds. SHAPER, A. G., HUTT, M. S. R. and FEJFAR, Z. London: British Medical Association.

STAMLER, J. J. (1967) *Lectures on Preventive Cardiology*. New York: Grune and Stratton.

TYROLER, H. A. and CASSEL, J. (1964) Health consequences of culture change. II. The effect of urbanization on coronary heart mortality in rural residents. *Journal of Chronic Diseases*, **17**, 167–177.

VAUGHAN, J. P. and MIALL, W. E. (1978) A comparison of cardiovascular measurements in The Gambia, Jamaica, and the United Republic of Tanzania. *Bulletin of the World Health Organization*, **57**, 281–289.

SOCIAL CLASS AND DISEASE

R. A. CARTWRIGHT

Yorkshire Regional Cancer Organisation, Cookridge Hospital, Leeds

OCCUPATION has been routinely recorded in England and Wales on death certificates and in the decennial Censuses since the mid 19th century. This was through the influence of medical statisticians such as William Farr (1864); these innovators viewed disease as a consequence to a greater or lesser extent of the social circumstances of the patient, which would, in turn, be an indication of the sum of the environmental experience that an individual had had up to the onset of the disease. Occupations were recorded in a fairly arbitrary fashion until the Census of 1911, when Stevenson, the Chief Medical Statistician, and successor of William Farr, introduced the concept that an ordinal measure of lifestyle could be devised. He termed this the social class scale and based it entirely on the occupation as recorded in the enumerators' returns for the Census. The original scale had five sub-divisions:

I	Professional
II	Intermediate
III	Skilled
IV	Semi-skilled
V	Unskilled

Later the skilled group was sub-divided into non-manual and manual sections (IIIN and IIIM) allowing broad manual/non-manual group analyses to be made. Many changes and refinements have been made to the classification with each Census, in particular in the scope and description of occupations. In parallel with the changes in concepts and compositions of these English social class tabulations, various other developments have gone on in relation to occupational categorization and sub-grouping. All these are summarized in the Classification of Occupation (1970); all other subdivisions are based on the 223 occupational units which can give the 27 occupational orders and the 17 socio-economic groups. These latter groups are a development since the 1940s of a new attempt to stratify occupations which would also be meaningful in social, cultural and recreational terms.

All the classes, groups and orders can be derived from the basic occupational units and these, in turn, need a clear and detailed job description from each individual. Little is said further about the uses of the occupational units, although the critique at the end of this chapter could equally apply to these newer divisions as well as to social class.

This evolution in the use of occupation as a basis for social classifications of this kind is almost unique to the United Kingdom, and has been developed in such a way along with the Standard Industrial Classification (1968) that international comparisons are difficult and probably meaningless. Insofar as our society is unique through its particular social, historical, economic and medical institutions, the lack of such international comparability is perhaps to be expected. Diseases at least have some international comparability through the efforts of the World Health Organization, which produces the decennial International Classification of Disease (World Health Organization, 1977). Even with diseases, however, there are many difficulties in interpretation, conceptualization and agreed comparison.

Classifications of social standards by routine data in other countries, where attempted, are based either on their own occupational spectra or on economic indices such as those used in the United States of America. Occasionally attempts at combining such factors as occupation and income have been made to produce indices which reflect more accurately the economic status and environmental lifestyle of each population sub-group.

Uses of social class in disease studies
The social class measure of Stevenson proved an immediate and lasting success, in that it demonstrated marked ordinal differences

between the sub-population with respect to a wide variety of disease indicators. The standardized mortality ratios, for example, for adult males dying before retirement had always had a trend to higher mortality in the 'lower' social classes, i.e., IV and V, and are summarized in Table 1. Before 1924 the data are given as Comparative Mortality Figures and after they are expressed as Standardized Mortality Ratio.

These trends are a constant feature of all social class statistics in relation to many aspects of society and have led to adoption of this description of social class as a measure of differences in disease patterns for every imaginable disease group in all types of special studies as well as in the analysis of routinely collected data. In addition, the relations between possible aetiological factors, either environmental or intrinsic, and social class have received increasing attention.

Secular trends in disease and social class within the UK have been successfully and consistently demonstrated, the work of Susser and Stein (1962) on trends in peptic ulceration with age, time and social class being a particularly clear example of this. Duodenal ulcers and gastric ulcers have been changing since the last century in terms of incidence, prevalence and their presenting features. The various factors were dissected out by cohort analysis and it became clear that in the 1920s there were no social class gradients for deaths from duodenal ulceration below the age of 45. However, this age group in successive decades not only produced very high mortality figures, but this mortality was disproportionately contributed to by the upper social classes, with successive age cohorts being less commonly

TABLE 1.   Mortality from all causes — standardized mortality rates.

| Time period | Social class | | | | |
	I	II	III	IV	V
1910–12	88	94	96	93	142
1921–23	82	94	95	101	125
1930–32	90	94	97	102	111
1949–53	98	94	101	94	118
1959–63	76	81	100	103	143
1970–72	77	81	104	114	137

affected and without the same social class gradient. Perhaps the upper social classes first felt the effects of a new set of environmental factors which then became distributed more equally through the other classes as time and economic circumstances changed. Thus the concept of duodenal ulceration being an upper social class disease is an historical one although still commonly held.

The same type of phenomenon has been investigated in arterial diseases, and here again the picture is not a simple one. Medical opinion and popular reports have long suggested a relationship between the arterial diseases and upper social classes. Yet Antonovsky (1968), in an exhaustive literature search, concluded that most studies where some form of social status was measured show a confused relationship between social class and the various arterial diseases. It was true to say, however, that almost all studies showed some sort of relationship. Again the situation is clarified by the examination of secular relationships. Early studies showed a clear social class gradient from the upper to the lower classes. Most studies since the 1950s, however, particularly in America, show no clear social gradient. The subject is confused by the lack of continuously monitored populations with clear definitions of arterial disease and accepted methods for defining morbidity and risk factors, in addition to all the problems of social class measurement which will be discussed later in the chapter.

Major contributions to disease studies with respect to social class and its uses have been made in relation to psychiatric disorders. Most psychiatric epidemiological studies have incorporated social class as a possible aetiological factor. Petras and Curtis (1968) review 350 studies for American populations alone. The work of Faris and Dunham (1939) showed that schizophrenics were found among the lowest social groups in the worst housing areas of Chicago, and they suggested that the appalling environmental surroundings there produced the disease. However, Goldberg and Morrison (1963), studying a series of consecutive admissions to one psychiatric unit in Britain, found that although the patients themselves were from the lower social classes, the pattern of social class in their parents was typical of the areas from which the patients originated. Downward social class movement had occurred in parallel with the onset of the disease but often preceded the clinical diagnosis; these results are shown in Table 2. This work has been confirmed and suggests that

TABLE 2.   Social class changes in schizophrenia.

Social class	% patient's father	% patient's at presentation	% patients 2–4 years later
I + II	29	15	2
III	48	40	29
IV	10	13	21
V	13	27	13
No occupation/unknown	0	4	35

adverse environmental influences are not aetiological but symptomatic for this particular sort of psychosis.

Studies on cancer are a good example of the commonly accepted ordinal relationship with social class, and these results are detailed in the recently published decennial supplement (*Occupational Mortality*, 1978) which analyses causes of death by occupational subgroups for the three years 1970–2. All cancers when aggregated together show a rise in the lower social classes and the results for men of working age are given in Table 3. However, the majority of male cancer deaths in this age group are due to the high prevalence of bronchus and

TABLE 3.   Standardized mortality ratio: social class and cancer 1970–72 men aged 15–64.

Social class	All cancers (ICD 140–209)	Stomach (151)	Lung and trachea (162)
I	75	50	53
II	80	66	68
IIIN	91	79	84
IIIM	113	118	118
IV	116	125	123
V	131	147	143

Social class	Intestine (152/153)	Leukaemias (204–7)
I	105	113
II	100	100
IIIN	105	107
IIIM	106	101
IV	101	104
V	109	95

stomach cancers and if these are removed, the aggregated results show less downward bias by social class. Some cancers have no social class bias, e.g., intestinal neoplasms, whilst others still seem to have a slight upper-class bias, as aggregated leukaemia deaths demonstrate. For 47 specific cancers there is a definite bias to the lower classes in 20, although the numbers of deaths in certain categories are very small. Of the remainder, there is an upper-class bias in 13 and the other 14 have indeterminate patterns—almost an equal distribution of the three possibilities, in fact.

In addition to the incidence of specific diseases, risk factors or determinants of disease can also be shown to vary with social class. Uric acid levels appear to vary with social class and thus may interact or confound in studies on gout and social class (Dunn et al., 1963). In addition it is possible that the ABO blood groups, which are associated specifically with some diseases (e.g., stomach cancer, duodenal ulceration and arterial diseases (Mourant, Kopeć and Domainiewska-Sobczak, 1978) may vary with social class. The following data are derived from a study which investigated this possibility.

Nearly 1000 blood donors from all parts of Nottingham City and the nearby coal-mining village of Edwinstowe were interviewed and their current occupation recorded. Blood samples were taken and tested for a variety of polymorphisms. The gene frequencies by social class are given in Table 4 (ABO: Cartwright and Hargreaves, unpublished; results for other systems have been published elsewhere: Cartwright, Hargreaves and Sunderland, 1978). Although there was no statistical heterogeneity between the social classes, some marked

TABLE 4.   Ranges of gene frequencies at seven loci.

Polymorphic genes	UK geographical data	Nottingham social class data
ABO (O gene)	0·05	0·04
Rh (d)	0·06	0·04
Haptoglobin 1 (Hp^1)	0·05	0·25
Transferrin C (Tf^c)	0·006	0·02
Acid phosphatase B (P^b)	0·05	0·08
Adenylate kinase 1 (AK^1)	0·02	0·01
Esterase D 1 (EsD^1)	0·07	0·04

differences in gene frequency by social class were shown by some polymorphisms, including the ABO system. It must be emphasized that whereas the geographical differences are statistically significant, much larger samples will be needed to give reliable estimates of interclass variation.

Because the blood groups have a range of associations with diseases (Mourant, Kopeć and Domaniewska-Sobczak, 1978), and as social class is also variable in a number of ways for the same diseases, these observations, if confirmed, could have far-reaching implications. Are the genetic relationships fortuitous or are they the cause of the primary observations on social classes in disease? Neither alternative sounds particularly attractive, and there is as yet no good evidence for either. Biological relationships in general tend to be more complex, however. Certainly, future studies based on sound epidemiological principles should be set up to examine prospectively an incident disease series and compare it with a large case-comparison group so that the possible interactive or confounding effects of genetic factors of all types could be related to social class.

In all the studies so far mentioned, it has been implicit that social class is as easy to define as the disease entity itself. In fact, neither are easily categorized. It is my contention that social class should not be taken as an easy and useful measure of lifestyle, but should be used with care, taking all its disadvantages into account. This might allow us to review the relationship of social class to disease more critically and suggest how future studies could be carried out.

Critique of Social Class in the United Kingdom

Every society has some type of social stratification within it. Within certain societies, e.g., some hunter–gatherer populations in Africa, roles are more or less clearly defined and few major changes are likely to have occurred for many generations. Similarly, historical populations in the United Kingdom have contained clearly stratified subgroups, which were quite well-defined, although allowing some mobility between them. Even by the mid 19th century, lifestyles were clearly enough defined and the social pattern was well enough set to allow various assumptions to be made, for example that income had a fixed relation to occupation, and that interoccupational mobility was sufficiently rare to be ignored. A given occupation allowed one to assume a great deal about the habits, economics, taste, housing, food, clothing, cleanliness, hobbies, alcohol consumption of the man and his family. To William Farr and his contemporaries, a population of printers, farriers or tailors could be well-defined in all these respects simply by a knowledge of the occupation of the head of the household. Similarly, the success in the early 20th century of the broader concepts of manual/non-manual, skilled, semi-skilled and unskilled, was due to the particular nature of our society at that time.

Is it possible to still accept these concepts upon which Stevenson based social class? Probably it is not, if we are to use social class as it was originally intended, as a convenient and useful measure of social stratification. The reasons for this are largely due to the rapidity with which social change has occurred within our society, in particular over the last four decades.

Employed women never properly fitted into the classification of Stevenson, for example the textile workers of Lancashire, and originally social class did not include women. The additional changes over the last few decades, leading in 1971 to 38 per cent of the economically active workforce being female, has been ignored in the general statistics unless the women were single. However, many married women might influence the total environmental circumstances of their households either for better or for worse with respect to disease; yet this possibility has been generally ignored. No studies appear to have investigated the possible role, if any, of such influences on arterial disease or cancers, nor have the overall relationships between occupation and disease in women been investigated effectively.

Intergenerational mobility must always have existed, even though no allowance was made for this possibility in the study of parental and offspring occupation groups of Goldberg and Morrison (1963) noted above, in common with most studies of that type. Work in Nottingham asking blood donors the social class of parents has revealed a complex set of changes which suggests that such factors ought to be taken into account in disease studies. Table 5 summarizes these results and shows that between two generations only a third of adults have the same social class as their parents. Thus social environments and the apparent risks of developing certain diseases have changed in an individual's lifetime.

Individual variation within social class groups within the person's own lifetime is not often discussed in the literature, but is of particular

TABLE 5. Social class intergenerational mobility in Nottingham.

	%
Up 5 classes	0·1
4	1·9
3	4·3
2	16·1
1	20·7
No change	36·6
Down 1 class	11·9
2	6·6
3	1·3
4	0·5
5	0

importance to epidemiologists. Cross-sectional studies such as the decennial Censuses only reveal one occupation per person, which might be transient or lifelong. Such within-individual variation must influence the total variance within the social class estimates. It is often argued that if a large population is studied, the associations revealed will of themselves be useful, but without hard data on contemporary social class mobility, this is difficult to accept.

A series of retired men from Bradford, selected at random from general practitioner lists, have had complete occupational interviews (Cartwright, unpublished). The overall distribution of numbers of different social classes is shown in Table 6 for the first hundred. There has been wide variation in the occupational histories of these men. This can be measured in three ways — by the different occupational descriptions of each man, by the number of different employers, (irrespective of occupational description) and finally by change of social class. Some men have only had one social class throughout

TABLE 6. Number of social classes per person (retired men in Bradford).

	%
1	20
2	37
3	34
4	8
5	1

their lives, but the majority have had several: an average of 2·3 social classes each. The mean number of different occupational descriptions experienced by the men is 3·7 and if one takes the number of jobs with different firms into account, each man has had on average 4·5 employers, although often he has done a similar type of job with different employers.

The distribution of social class within this population over time is thus difficult to interpret; Table 7 shows the overall social class score distribution, taking at least one different score per individual, together with the scores at retirement. There is no obvious bias here between lifetime experience and final social class. This is an important point, because a great deal of the routinely collected mortality data relies on the last occupation in retired or chronically sick individuals. The overall results differ somewhat from the Censuses of 1961 and 1971, and this reflects regional trends in social class. Such local trends have been routinely documented and interpreted as accounting for patterns of disease mortality such as those presented by Howe (1970).

Those with one lifetime social class are distributed mainly in classes IIIM or IV with only one person each in classes II and IIIN. This presentation of data reveals little of the true situation, and if the results are taken as ordinal events occurring over time, a complex pattern of change is seen, with a minority of individuals (20 per cent) exhibiting no social class change throughout their lives, whilst others move up and down the scale several times. Table 8 summarizes the major individual social class variation, expressed as the maximum amount of change experienced by one person in his working life.

TABLE 7.   Social class histories.

	Bradford total class distribution (%)	Bradford classes at retirement (%)	Census 1961 England and Wales (%)	1971 (%)
I	0·9	1·0	2·9	4·8
II	10·0	13·0	15·5	19·9
IIIN	12·1 } 46·7	10·0 } 46·1	51·0	16·0 } 49·0
IIIM	34·6	36·0		33·0
IV	32·9	35·0	23·1	18·7
V	9·5	5·0	8·5	7·6

TABLE 8.   Maximum changes in social class in one generation (Bradford data).

	%
Up 4 classes	2
3	6
2	15
1	23
No class change	20
Down 1 class	18
2	8
3	8

If social class is to be meaningful in disease studies, especially for the common chronic diseases such as the arterial disorders and the cancers, then it is necessary that social class reflect the lifestyle of the individual. If the data given above are representative, then this is manifestly not the case.

Secular trends are often computed on social class and disease. A few have been detailed earlier, and yet it is often implied in many of these studies that the natural history of the disease can change while the social classes remain stable. This is not the case individually and because of change in the occupational classification codes, in job description and in the nature of jobs, social class itself must be in all aspects as prone to secular change as the diseases under study.

Thus various practical difficulties emerge with respect to social class interpretation. These also extend to the methodology of data collection. Does one collect individual information upon the longest particular occupation a workman has had and use that for the social class estimate? The Bradford data suggest this would be difficult if one is to use the concept fully. Unfortunately, code modification would allow misinterpretation and bias to enter the study. For example, the spectra of occupations in bladder cancer cases would be biased away from risk occupation if they were selected on length of occupation, as evidence suggests that carcinogenic exposure of less than a year is sufficient to produce this cancer often decades later. Similarly at the social class level, a class which might mean exposure to hazardous substances could be ignored. Should one then take into account all social classes to the time of the onset of the disease and monitor further classes until death? This is rarely, if ever, done and yet seems to be the only unbiased way of fairly assessing occupational and class risks in disease.

This approach produces further problems, however, including those of getting sufficient detail in historical terms to allow accurate social class interpretation to be made. Again, should one use the contemporary coding system for that period or try to apply the most modern system? The difficulties individuals have of recalling their working histories must lead to errors, and the significance of such errors is currently being investigated by the author.

Thus we may conclude that social class should not be taken as an immutable concept with which to study disease; it changes with time, and in the individual, and does not form the basis for good quality data.

Some of the largest changes in our rapidly changing society have occurred in the field of pay differentials, job types and the working conditions in many common occupations. None of these are directly accounted for by social class. Ineichen (1972), for example, has shown that lifestyles of manual workers in Bristol differ according to the type of home accommodation, and this often applies to men in the same kind of work. Social classes as individual occupations or groups of occupation now have a wide range of possible environmental experiences, something not at all anticipated by Farr or Stevenson. Even one and a half decades ago, Goldthorpe (1970) found no such inter-occupational variation. Nowadays, however, we ought to take more account of studies on variation in the social life of members of each class and the way this influences disease patterns.

A few decades ago, social strata carried sufficient of the status ethic of that group to allow meaningful behavioural distinctions to be made. This has changed. Carcinoma of the cervix provides a good example of the misinterpretation now inherent in social class which was probably not present (although admittedly not looked for) some years ago. When the rates are based on husband's occupation, carcinoma of the cervix is more common in the lower social classes. However, Table 9 shows that within each class, the rates for the minimally and maximally affected groups vary considerably and that the 'high risk' male occupations are often shift workers. This could allow more sexual freedom among their wives.

Nowadays, economic, social, cultural and other behavioural patterns cut across the social classes in a way which not even the more

TABLE 9. Occupational subgroups by social class: SMR for carcinoma of the cervix by occupation of the husband.

		SMR		SMR
I	Clergymen	12	Civil engineers	60
II	Local government officers	18	Aircraft pilots	150
IIIN	Secretaries	33	Policemen	138
IIIM	Printers	21	Coal-miners	197
IV	Agricultural drivers	25	Seamen	263
V	Cleaners	95	Gas works labourers	229

modern groupings of occupation nor a computation based on family income can unravel. If particular diseases are due to some aspect of lifestyle other than occupation, as is often likely to be the case, then such routinely collected measures as are commonly available — age, place of residence, occupation, and income — are completely inadequate. New measures are required to tell us of possible carcinogenic exposure throughout a person's life: smoking and alcohol experience, atmospheric pollution, home circumstances, contact with animals, exercise, sexual activities and diet. Diet, in particular, is of such importance as to require very detailed analysis. These particular aspects of lifestyle cover only a few of the known or assumed risks in arterial, chest and neoplastic diseases. If the search is for new aetiological agents or factors which influence disease, the study of routinely collected social class statistics or even special prospective studies can do nothing but indicate very crude relationships and only then if the underlying factors strongly influence the disease. Weak associations would be lost within the intraoccupation–class variation.

Even if the diseases under investigation have an occupational element, social class status is a redundant and even confusing measure to use because of occupational changes and difficulties in recording the data. In addition, people move from job to job of the same type, but in different firms with often very different working conditions; large corporations are safety-conscious and allow little chemical exposure to the work-force, but this is often not the case with small or medium-sized firms where conditions are lax and the work-force continually changing. Again, workmen can stay in one firm but be engaged in a number of jobs, each with different hazards. Finally, the same job within the same firm can change over the years to be more or less hazardous as new techniques are introduced. Social class takes little account of these differences.

References

ANTONOVSKY, A. (1968) Social class and the major cardiovascular diseases. *Journal of Chronic Diseases,* **21,** 65–106.

CARTWRIGHT, R. A., HARGREAVES, H. J. and SUNDERLAND, E. (1978) Social identity and genetic variability. *Journal of Biosocial Science,* **10,** 23–33.

Classification of Occupation 1970. O.P.C.S. (1920). London: H.M.S.O.

DUNN, J. P., BROOKS, G. W., MAUSNER, J., RODNAM, G. P. and COBB, S. (1963) Social class gradient and serum uric acid levels in males. *Journal of the American Medical Association,* **185,** 431–6.

FARIS, R. E. L. and DUNHAM, H. W. (1939) *Mental Disorders in Urban Areas.* Chicago: University of Chicago Press.

FARR, W. (1864) *Letter to the Registrar General in Supplement to the 25th Annual Report of the Registrar General of Births, Death and Marriages in England,* pp. xxxv–xxxvi and p. 440. London: H.M.S.O.

GOLDBERG, E. M. and MORRISON, S. L. (1963) Schizophrenia and social class. *British Journal of Psychiatry,* **109,** 785.

GOLDTHORPE, J. H. (1970) L'image des classes chez les travailleurs manuels aisés. *Revue Français de Sociologie,* **11,** 311–338.

HOWE, G. M. (1970) *National Atlas of Disease Mortality in the United Kingdom.* London: Nelson.

INEICHEN, B. (1972) Home ownership and manual working lifestyles. *Sociology Review,* **20,** (n.s.) 391–412.

MOURANT, A. E., KOPEĆ, A. C. and DOMANIEWSKA-SOBCZAK, K. (1978) *Blood Groups and Diseases.* Oxford: Oxford University Press.

Occupational Mortality 1970-72. (1978) England and Wales Decennial Supplement. O.P.C.S. London: H.M.S.O.

PETRAS, H. W. and CURTIS, J. E. (1968) The current literature on social class and mental disease in America: critique and bibliography. *Behavioural Science,* **13,** 382-98.

STEVENSON, T. H. C. (1923) The social distribution of mortality in England and Wales 1910–1912. *Biometrika,* **15,** 382–400.

SUSSER, M. W. and STEIN, Z. A. (1962) Civilization and peptic ulcer. *Lancet,* **i,** 115–9.

WORLD HEALTH ORGANIZATION (1977) *International Classification of Disease,* 9th edn. Geneva: World Health Organization.

AUTHOR INDEX

SUBJECT INDEX

Printed and bound by CPI Group (UK) Ltd, Croydon, CR0 4YY

17/10/2024

01775680-0008